EPILEPSY

Clearly describes the basic facts about this condition, explaining the medical aspects in understandable terms, and providing practical advice to help overcome the problems.

D0586968

EPILEPSY

What it is, what causes it and advice on its successful management

by

Peter Hazeldine

THORSONS PUBLISHING GROUP
Wellingborough, Northamptonshire
Rochester, Vermont

First published 1986
Second Impression 1987

British Library Cataloguing in Publication Data

Hazeldine, Peter
    Epilepsy: what it is, what causes it and advice
    on its successful management.
    1. Epilepsy
    I. Title
    616.8'53   RC372

    ISBN 0-7225-1249 X

Printed and bound in Great Britain

CONTENTS

FOREWORD

Over the past few years there has been a considerable increase in the number of books on epilepsy. In itself, this is indicative of a growing awareness of the condition, and a need for information through the printed word.

Although epilepsy is primarily a medical phenomenon, those who live with it frequently suffer more from public attitudes than from the epilepsy. It is not an exaggeration to say that the stigma of epilepsy still exists in this modern age.

Peter Hazeldine's book is completely comprehensive in its examination of both the medical and social aspects of epilepsy. This book is a veritable fund of facts and will be of great value to professional and lay people alike, to those who have epilepsy and to those who do not. It is one more significant milestone on the road to a clearer understanding of a condition which, for many generations, has been grossly misunderstood.

ALEC ASPINALL,
Chief Executive,
British Epilepsy Association,
Leeds.

INTRODUCTION

At least one person in every two hundred has epilepsy (possibly one in every hundred). Even on a conservative estimate there are well over 300,000 epileptics in Britain today, and each year a further 30-40,000 new cases are diagnosed.

Epilepsy is a very old disease. It is mentioned in the Code of Hammurabi, written some 4,000 years ago, and it is the subject of the earliest work of scientific medicine to survive, *The Sacred Disease,* attributed to the Greek physician Hippocrates. Over the centuries epileptic seizures have been variously explained as a form of spirit possession, as a punishment for sin, as a contagion spread on the patient's breath, and as a type of madness.

Many people have epilepsy, but only a few have such poor seizure-control as to be recognizable as epileptic; yet it is on this small and unrepresentative group that stereotypes about epilepsy tend to be based. Ancient superstitions have not faded away; they have merely been transformed. To judge from the results of surveys carried out here and in the USA, the public-at-large still think of the 'typical epileptic' as a shy, sluggish, mentally-retarded soul, given to occasional bouts of purposeless violence, and of epilepsy as a disorder which patients 'suffer from' and are 'afflicted by'. In reality, people with epilepsy frequently suffer more from the effects of prejudice than they do from their own fits. Epilepsy is not the crippling disease it is so often thought to be. Seizures can be coped with.

I say this with some feeling. It is now over twenty-five years since I had my first epileptic seizure: I was twelve at the time. Lately, my fits have been well-controlled. I possess a driving licence, I go swimming, I travel abroad; in fact, I do most of the things I would probably do if I didn't have epilepsy. I am fortunate in this respect, but I am not unique. There are many people who could tell the same story.

My hope is that what I have written will be of some benefit to patients, to their families and friends, to social workers, teachers and nurses, and to anyone wishing to learn about this complex and fascinating condition. I am not medically-trained, but I have read widely in the literature of epilepsy, and as a lay person I believe I am in a position to understand what lay people require from a book like this.

Finally, a word about language: I use *seizure* and *fit* interchangeably in the book to describe any kind of epileptic attack; *convulsion* I reserve for those kind of fits that involve the muscles; however, I make no distinction between anticonvulsant drugs and anti-epileptic drugs. Anticonvulsants are simply drugs that control seizures. For the sake of brevity, I often refer to people with epilepsy as epileptics or patients, although I realize that the term epileptic has a slightly institutionalized odour about it, and that, properly-speaking, epileptics are only patients when they are undergoing treatment.

1.

WHAT IS EPILEPSY?

People with epilepsy have fits or seizures, caused by sudden disturbances in the normal functioning of the brain. Epilepsy is not a fatal disease, nor is it a form of madness. Although some people with epilepsy have personality problems or are mentally retarded, the majority of patients live normal lives, their seizures well-controlled by medication.

The word epilepsy is derived from the Greek, *epilambaneia,* which means 'to seize, to take hold of'. It was originally used in connection with one particular kind of fit, what we now call grand mal, or — to give it its proper name — generalized tonic-clonic epilepsy, in which the patient loses consciousness, sinks to the ground and has convulsions. Many people still think of epilepsy in terms of the grand mal fit without realizing that there are other kinds of seizures as well. For example, some patients have convulsions down only one side of the body, or in a finger, or at the side of the mouth. Others have no convulsions at all, but merely stare vacantly for a second or two, or smack their lips, or hallucinate, or experience intense feelings of dread and despair.

Epilepsy is a symptom of many different diseases, not a disease in its own right. The difference is important. Influenza, for instance, is a disease, but a high temperature, a runny nose and stiffness in the joints — these are all symptoms. When we are ill, the first thing we want is some relief from our symptoms, from the pain, or the fever, or the nausea that is causing us such distress; but we also hope that the underlying cause of our illness can be discovered and cured. In the case of epilepsy, the underlying causes are often unknown and incurable. Treatment of epilepsy is almost exclusively a matter of dealing with the symptoms — of controlling the seizures.

A single, isolated fit is never, by itself, sufficient proof of epilepsy.

Young babies are especially prone to convulsions when they are feverish, but in most cases their seizures do not return after the illness that provoked them has been overcome. It is only when fits are recurrent, and when they take one of several characteristic forms, that epilepsy can be suspected; and even then a doctor will usually require additional evidence before reaching a final diagnosis.

What all epileptic seizures have in common is that they originate in the brain, or — to be more precise — in the central nervous system, of which the brain is the superior part, the headquarters. The fact that everyone has a brain means we are all, without exception, susceptible to fits. In this one respect epilepsy is rather akin to pain. We can all feel pain, but some people are more sensitive to it than others. This is not because they are weaker than anyone else, but simply because that is the way they are made. Such people are born, as we say, with a low pain threshold. It is the same with epilepsy. Anyone can have a seizure, although only certain people do — they have a low *seizure* threshold. The treatment of epilepsy usually consists of the administration of special drugs that raise this threshold to a more normal level.

Since epilepsy is caused by disturbances in the brain, it is to the brain we must first look in order to understand what epilepsy is.

The Nerve Cell

The central nervous system is composed of two kinds of cells: the nerve cell, or *neuron,* and the *glia* cell. The job of the neuron is to transmit the nerve messages that activate the various parts of the body. The smaller, but more numerous glia are the soil in which the neurons are planted. They provide the neurons with mechanical support, nourishment, and protection against injury.

Nerve messages take the form of electro-chemical signals. These are sent off, one at a time, like a rapid pulse, whenever a neuron discharges, or fires. *Sensory* impulses travel from the sense organs to the brain and keep the brain informed of what is happening around it, in the body and in the outside world. *Motor* impulses travel from the brain to the muscles and tell the muscles when to move and when to stop moving.

Figure 1 illustrates the basic structure of the neuron. At its centre is a dark mass, the *nucleus,* that contains the genetic material the cell uses to repair itself. A thin envelope, the *membrane,* surrounds the neuron and from its surface sprouts a forest of stalk-like objects.

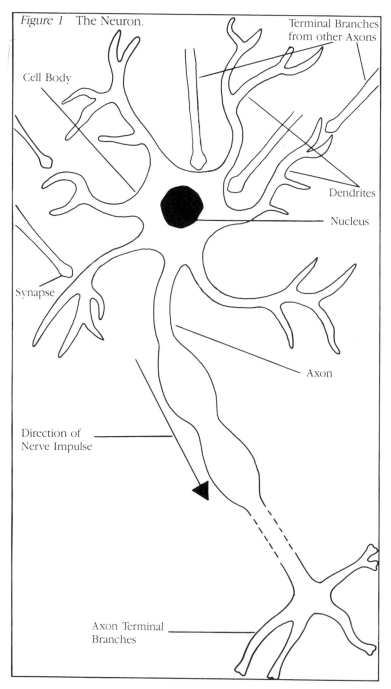

Figure 1   The Neuron.

Terminal Branches from other Axons

Cell Body

Dendrites

Nucleus

Synapse

Axon

Direction of Nerve Impulse

Axon Terminal Branches

These are of two kinds: *axons* and *dendrites*. The nerve impulse is carried *away* from the neuron along the axon and *to* the neuron along the dendrites. Each neuron has one axon and about 20,000 dendrites. What are popularly called nerves are really large bundles of axons bound together by connective tissue and wrapped in a fatty sheaf. The sheaf acts as a kind of insulator, like the rubber round an electric cable.

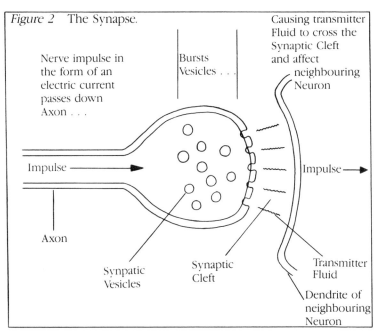

Figure 2   The Synapse.

Nerve impulse in the form of an electric current passes down Axon . . .

Bursts Vesicles . . .

Causing transmitter Fluid to cross the Synaptic Cleft and affect neighbouring Neuron

Impulse →

Impulse →

Axon

Synaptic Vesicles

Synaptic Cleft

Transmitter Fluid

Dendrite of neighbouring Neuron

The Nerve Impulse

Both the neuron and the fluid in which it bathes contain molecules that carry an electric charge: these are called *ions*. The rate at which ions enter and leave the neuron is controlled by the pump-like action of the membrane. Under certain conditions (to be described below) the membrane pump shuts down and a more rapid exchange of ions takes place. This in turn generates an electric current, which then travels down the whole length of the axon, in a succession of jumps, at a speed of between twenty-five and forty metres a second. Once the current has passed, the membrane pump starts up again, the excess ions are expelled and the neuron returns to its resting state.

Neurons are not physically connected to one another. Between a neuron and its neighbour is a minute gap, the *synapse* (see Figure

2). At the end of the axon is a collection of small bag-like objects called *vesicles,* each one of which contains a type of chemical known as a *transmitter substance,* or *neurotransmitter.* The nerve impulse, as it reaches the end of the axon, punctures some of the vesicles, and the transmitter substance flows out across the synapse, where it comes into contact with the membrane of a neighbouring neuron.

What happens next depends on whether the neurotransmitter is an *excitatory* or an *inhibitory* one. Excitatory neurotransmitters stimulate the neurons into discharging by slowing down the action of the membrane pump. Inhibitory neurotransmitters have the opposite effect. By strengthening the action of the membrane pump they reduce the exchange of ions and so retard the neurons from firing. At any one time, a neuron is receiving, by way of its dendrites, messages from thousands of other neurons, some of which are excitatory and some inhibitory. Whether or not a neuron eventually fires depends on which of the two competing sets of messages are in the majority — a very democratic arrangement.

Reflex Actions

If you gently touch an earthworm with a stick, it will automatically curl up. This is an example of a *reflex action.* The sensory stimulus (the touch of the stick) is immediately converted into a muscular response (the body curls up). Reflexes are organized in the spinal cord, not in the brain. They are the most basic form of all nervous activity, but they have been retained throughout evolution because they provide a quick and decisive way of responding to danger. It is, for example, a reflex action that makes us withdraw our hand as soon as it touches a hot object. The sensory stimulus takes longer to reach the brain than it does the spinal cord, and that is why, by the time we feel the pain caused by the burn, our hand has already been withdrawn.

Because it has only a rudimentary nervous system, the earthworm is very much a prey to its own reflexes. Once a stimulus has reached a certain intensity, it cannot help but react. The same is not true for human beings. Our nervous system contains numerous synapses which, by exerting a modifying influence over the neurons, serve to inhibit responses. Thanks to the synapses we are able to do what earthworms cannot, i.e. we can override our reflexes and make considered decisions on how to behave.

The Epileptic Focus

Epileptic seizures often (perhaps always) start from around the site of an injury. There are many ways in which the brain can be injured — blows to the head, tumours, infections and so on — but the end result is the same each time. At the spot where the injury occurs, the neurons are destroyed. Close by they remain functioning, but crippled. The site from which a seizure originates — the *epileptic focus* — is composed of such crippled, poorly-functioning neurons. Lacking the normal powers of inhibition, neurons within a focus tend to be electrically very unstable. What would otherwise be a short-lived neural impulse may, if it is generated within a focus, develop unchecked and begin to exert an influence over more and more distant areas. It is not possible to say for certain that all seizures are the result of a failure in inhibition. Some fits are probably caused by stimuli which are so strong that no brain could resist them. Fits induced by electro-therapy, or by certain drugs, are a case in point. But many *epileptic* seizures are undoubtedly due to under-inhibition rather than over-excitation.

The Seizure Discharge

The activity of a single neuron is too feeble to have any appreciable effect on the brain as a whole. Neurons, however, are organized into groups consisting of several hundreds of thousands of members. At any one time some of the neurons in a group will be firing, others will be recovering after having fired, and others will be resting, primed to fire. Because of the deficency of their inhibitory controls, neurons in an epileptic focus tend to discharge together, as a single unit. In terms of numbers, such neurons may represent only a small part of a cell group; nevertheless, when they do discharge, their combined electrical output may be many times greater than that of all the other neurons in the group, only a proportion of which are firing at any one time. An impulse generated in a focus may thus be sufficiently powerful to overlap into an adjacent group of neurons and to stimulate them into firing. This group in turn may set off a third, and so on, like a line of dominoes falling over. The result is a *seizure discharge;* a neural impulse that rapidly runs out of control and causes such disruption to normal brain activity that a fit develops.

All epileptic fits begin in this way, with a seizure discharge, but the symptoms of a fit depend on the area in the brain in which the seizure discharge takes place. This will become clearer if we look at the structure of the brain.

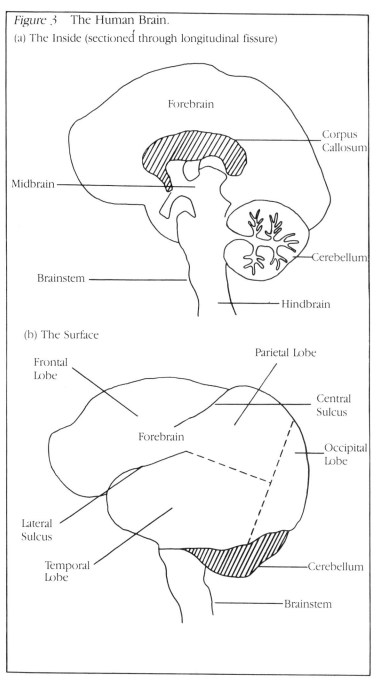

Figure 3 The Human Brain.

(a) The Inside (sectioned through longitudinal fissure)

(b) The Surface

The Brain

The human brain (see Figure 3) is like a house three storeys high. The ground floor is the *hindbrain*. It is from here that breathing, digestion and excretion, functions essential for the maintenance of life, are controlled. The hindbrain is a robust structure; it has changed little in the course of evolution and is not affected by the explosive discharges that cause fits.

Next, a storey higher, comes the *midbrain,* which together with the hindbrain, forms the *brainstem*. Modifications in our level of awareness are regulated by the midbrain, as too are the rhythms of sleep and waking.

Behind the brainstem lies the *cerebellum,* a vaguely spherical organ, about the size of a tangerine. The function of the cerebellum is to maintain balance and co-ordination, a task it achieves by filtering out the neural impulses despatched to the muscles from the forebrain (see below). People who have suffered damage to the cerebellum have great difficulty in picking up small objects and are often unsteady on their feet, especially when walking.

Although certain types of generalized fits originate in the midbrain, most seizure discharges take place in the highest, most complex and, for that reason, most easily disturbed level of the brain — the *forebrain.*

The Forebrain

The forebrain (see Figure 4) is divided into two equal halves, the *right* and *left cerebral hemispheres,* by a groove called the *longitudinal fissure.* Broadly speaking, our analytical skills, including the understanding and articulation of language, are organized in the left, or dominant, hemisphere, while the right hemisphere is more concerned with the organization of spatial skills of the kind that allow us to recognize faces and orientate ourselves in space. The two hemispheres are connected by several tracts of nerve fibres, the most important of which, made up of about 100 million axons, is the *corpus callosum.* The messages that pass backwards and forwards along these nerve tracts ensure that the two hemispheres remain in constant contact with each other.

All the higher intellectual processes are organized within the *cerebral cortex,* a sheet of neurons about one-tenth of an inch (2mm) thick, enveloping the entire surface of the forebrain. Because it is so rucked-up and wrinkled, the cerebral cortex looks

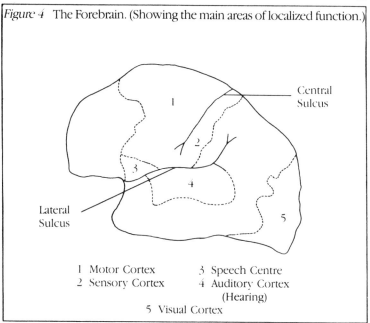

Figure 4 The Forebrain. (Showing the main areas of localized function.)

Central Sulcus

Lateral Sulcus

1 Motor Cortex   3 Speech Centre
2 Sensory Cortex   4 Auditory Cortex
(Hearing)
5 Visual Cortex

smaller than it is; laid out flat it would cover an area of about three square feet. The grooves, or fissures, in the cortex are known as *sulci.* Two of the most important sulci (the *lateral* and *central sulci*) cross to form the boundary lines between the four *lobes:* the *frontal, parietal, occipital* and *temporal.* Of these, it is the temporal lobes (there is one in each hemisphere) we shall encounter most often in this book. Within them are to be found the areas where sounds, tastes and smells are interpreted, as well as other zones associated with the faculties of memory and emotion that are particularly susceptible to the effects of a seizure discharge. Injury to the temporal lobes is one of the commonest known causes of epilepsy.

Although memory is partly dependent on the proper functioning of the temporal lobes, there is no single memory centre as such in the brain. Like thinking, imagination and the other higher faculties (excluding language), what we call memory is really the end-product of the co-ordinated activity of many different parts of the brain. Some of the simpler faculties, however, are run from specific brain centres. Among the most important of these centres are the *motor cortex,* where voluntary movements are organized, and the *sensory cortex,* where the nerve messages from the surface layers of the body are received and interpreted.

Movement and Sensation

The motor cortex is situated in front of the central sulcus, over both hemisheres. Muscles on the right-hand side of the body are controlled by neurons in the left motor cortex; the neurons in the right motor cortex control the muscles on the left-hand side of the body. Thus, whenever a patient has a convulsion in, say, the left arm, we can be sure that the seizure discharge is taking place in the right side of the brain. The motor cortex is laid out in a precise way, with the neurons responsible for the feet and legs at the top, followed in descending order by the neurons for the shoulders, arms, hands, eyelids, lips and jaws. Those parts of the body, such as the fingers, which are called on to perform finely-graded movements are linked to more neurons than are those parts with only a limited range of movements, such as the biceps.

At the risk of oversimplifying what is in reality a complex system, we can compare the relationship between the neurons in the motor cortex and the voluntary muscles (muscles over which we have no direct control, like the heart, are connected to different parts of the brain) with that which exists between the keys on a piano and the notes they play. Each key sounds only one note, just as each group of neurons controls only one muscle. A seizure discharge is like a wild arpeggio. It sweeps through the motor cortex like a hand running along a keyboard causing successive groups of neurons (keys) to discharge (play) and successive groups of muscles (notes) to convulse (sound). Often this happens so quickly that a large number of muscles begin to convulse more or less at the same instant; but in certain cases of focal epilepsy, where a seizure discharge spreads more slowly, it is possible to observe its effects on the motor cortex as first one set of muscles, then a second, then a third begin to convulse — the convulsions radiating out over a wider and wider area in a systematic way.

Directly behind the motor cortex, and closely linked with it, is the sensory cortex. This is laid out in a similar fashion to the motor cortex, with the neurons for the feet and legs at the top and those for the face at the bottom. Areas of special sensitivity, such as the fingertips, lips and tongue are connected to a far greater number of neurons than are more insensitive areas, such as the soles of the feet. The nerve fibres cross over as they enter the brain so that the sense receptors in the left-hand side of the body transmit their messages to the sensory cortex on the right side of the brain; and vice-versa. A seizure discharge in the sensory cortex produces sensations that appear to arise in the parts of the body linked to the neurons affected. So, when a seizure discharge disrupts the neurons which receive messages from the fingers, the patient feels a tingling in the fingers, or some similar, localized sensation. The fingers themselves, however, are not involved — only the brain is.

Centres which receive impulses from the other sense organs, including the eyes and the ears, also exist within the forebrain. A seizure discharge in the optical cortex, situated in the occipital lobes, results in the patient 'seeing' flashing lights or spots of colour; a seizure discharge in the auditory cortex, situated in the temporal lobes, results in the patient 'hearing' buzzing or humming sounds; and if the organs responsible for the processes of memory are likewise disturbed, a complex sensory seizure, in which the patient hallucinates actual scenes and people, may develop.

The Path of the Seizure Discharge

Depending on where it begins and how powerful it is, a seizure discharge can spread from a focus in one of three ways (see Figure 5):

— A seizure discharge orginating in the midbrain can spread upwards and outwards into both cerebral hemispheres at the same time, causing an immediate loss of consciousness. If the motor cortex is involved, convulsions will occur on both sides of the body. Fits of this nature are said to be *primary generalized.*

— A seizure discharge can remain confined to one cerebral hemisphere. The patient may have either motor or sensory seizures, or both, but will not lose consciousness. This kind of fit is known as a *focal,* or a *partial,* one.

— A seizure discharge that begins focally can spread from one cerebral hemisphere into the other, along the corpus collosum, or through the midbrain, and become *secondary generalized.* In a typical case, a patient may experience an hallucination (an *aura*) arising from a small part of one of the cerebral hemispheres; then, as the seizure becomes generalized, both sides of the patient's body start to convulse and consciousness is lost.

A seizure discharge always spreads along a preferred pathway, rather in the way that a piece of wood will crack along a line of fracture, or a stream will follow a furrow in the earth. As each

Figure 5   The three ways in which a seizure discharge can spread.

1 *Primary Generalized*   The seizure discharge arising from an epileptic focus (a) spreads into both cerebral hemispheres simultaneously. The patient loses consciousness.

2 *Focal*   The seizure discharge arising from an epileptic focus (b) remains confined to the cerebral hemisphere in which it begins. The patient remains partly conscious.

3 *Secondary Generalized*   The seizure discharge arising from an epileptic focus (b) in one cerebral hemisphere spreads into the other cerebral hemisphere. The patient loses consciousness.

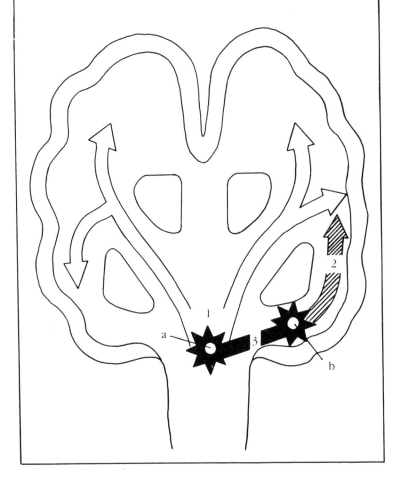

patient has only one preferred pathway in their brain, their fits will take the same form everytime.

Summary

Epilepsy is a symptom not a disease. What all epileptic fits have in common is that they are recurrent and that they are caused by an excessive and rapidly-spreading discharge of neurons in the brain: the so-called seizure discharge. The type of fit a person has depends on the area of the brain affected by the seizure discharge. Fits are basically of two kinds: generalized fits, where the seizure discharge disrupts both cerebral hemispheres and causes loss of consciouness; and focal or partial fits, in which only one cerebral hemisphere is disrupted and in which some degree of consciousness is retained.

2.

THE SYMPTOMS OF EPILEPSY

Generalized Seizures

Tonic-clonic seizures

Better known by the name of grand mal fits, these are the most easily recognizable, although not the commonest, form of epilepsy. About half of all cases begin with a type of partial seizure known as an *aura,* during which patients see flashing lights, hear a buzzing in their ears, experience strange tastes and smells, feel anxious, fluttering sensations in the abdomen, or have sudden, irrational fears. The precise symptom depends on the area of the brain affected by the seizure discharge. Although, strictly speaking, an aura represents the first stage of a fit, its appearance sometimes acts as a warning of an impending generalized seizure and gives the patient time to take precautionary measures, such as lying down, loosening tight-fitting clothes or removing dentures. At other times, the aura may be so brief that it is followed almost instantly by loss of consciousness.

The seizure discharge that creates the tonic-clonic fit disrupts the motor cortex over both hemispheres and causes the muscles to go into a spasm more or less at the same moment as consciousness is lost. A contracted muscle is described as being in a state of *tonus* (from the Greek word *tonos,* 'tension'), and the first stage of a grand mal fit, during which tonus persists, is called the *tonic stage.*

The sudden contraction or stiffening of the limbs at the start of the fit causes the patient to fall down, and the sudden contraction of the chest muscles forces air out of the lungs. So long as the muscles remain contracted, the lungs cannot reinflate and the patient is unable to breathe. His face turns blue-grey in colour from lack of oxygen and the veins stand out in his neck and forehead. Before falling to the ground, some patients emit a gurgling or strangled cry. If, however, the vocal cords go into a spasm at the same moment as the air expelled from the lungs is passing over them the cry will, in the manner of a bow being dragged across a taut violin string, take the form of a high-pitched scream, a sound so unlike the patient's normal voice that someone hearing it for the first time might well imagine the patient is in pain. This is not the case. The patient has already lost consciousness and the cry is purely an involuntary response. *At no time during a generalized seizure is the patient ever in pain.*

The body becomes starved of oxygen as the fit continues and this, in its turn, causes various physiological changes to take place that finally bring the tonic stage to a natural end after about twenty or thirty seconds. Momentarily, the muscles relax and air rushes into the lungs. The second, or *clonic,* stage of the fit now begins (*clonus* comes from a Greek word meaning 'violent motion'). The muscles alternately contract and relax, a process that at first causes the limbs to tremble and then, as the contractions grow further and further apart, to jerk violently. Some patients, especially the very young and the old, fracture a limb during the clonic stage of the fit, or become incontinent, voiding urine and occasionally faeces as bladder and bowels relax. Many patients bite the sides of their tongues, either at the start of the fit, when the jaws first snap shut, or later, during the clonic stage. Also a few, probably not as many as is popularly thought, drool from the mouth or nose. If the saliva becomes mixed with air from the lungs, a foam develops round the lips, and if the tongue is bitten this foam will be flecked with blood.

After about two minutes, the convulsions come to an end and the patient gradually returns to full consciousness. Patients are usually able to stand unsupported within about five minutes, although they will feel drained of strength for some while longer and may well want to sleep. It is not unusual for a patient to complain of a headache or of muscular stiffness following a fit, and some people — children mainly — suffer from a paralysis down one side of the body, known as *Todd's paresis,* that lasts for up to thirty-six hours. Sometimes, a fit is followed by a long period of confusion, aptly named a *twilight state,* during which the patient acts in a clumsy, drunken manner, becoming violent if any attempts are made to restrain him.

Clonic and myoclonic seizures

Myoclonic spasms are sudden, shock-like muscular jerks. They are not, in themselves, a sign of epilepsy. About 80 per cent of the adult population are subject to occasional bouts of *nocturnal myoclonus*. These usually occur at the beginning of sleep or immediately before waking, and take the form of a quick, convulsive kick, often accompanied or preceeded by a sensation of falling. Such spasms are a sign that the seizure threshold is at its lowest during sleep; however, not until such attacks begin to assume a more violent and repetitive form is it proper to consider them as a symptom of epilepsy.

A myoclonic seizure can be either generalized or focal and may consist of a single, explosive jerk or a sequence of such jerks. The seizure may be as mild as a nervous tic or it may be violent enough to throw a person to the ground. Sometimes it is the only epileptic symptom; often it accompanies other forms of seizure activity, such as absences, and it may, if it spreads, develop into a full-blown tonic-clonic convulsion. Any age group can be affected, although most patients are children.

West's syndrome, also known as *infantile spasms,* is a type of myoclonic epilepsy specific to new-born, brain-damaged children. The convulsions can take different forms. The body can be flexed upwards (a *jackknife attack*); the arms can be flung outwards (a *salaam attack*); or the head can nod towards the chest. These symptoms, which often occur in clusters, several times a day, take place against a background of general restlessness and are often accompanied by sudden cries.

The *Lennox-Gastaut syndrome* is found among older children, from about the age of four onwards. The convulsions are generalized and often violent, and patients sometimes injure themselves in falling. Some blurring of awareness may be caused and educational and emotional problems are common.

Familial myoclonic epilepsy is the result of a genetic defect that manifests itself in childhood or in early adulthood. Over the years, the myoclonic spasms develop into generalized tonic-clonic seizures and the patient's mental condition gradually deteriorates. Fortunately, this is a rare condition.

Absence seizures

Absence, or *petit mal,* seizures — to give them their more familiar name — are of two distinct kinds: *typical* and *atypical.* Typical absences are primary generalized. Atypical absences are secondary generalized.

A typical absence seizure takes the form of a sudden and brief loss of consciousness unaccompanied by muscular convulsions.

The patient stares vacantly, his face grows pale, his eyelids flicker and, so long as the fit lasts, he remains unresponsive to his surroundings. If he is speaking at the time the fit strikes, he will stop in mid-sentence, but he may continue to perform any task of a repetitive nature. Much depends on the depth and duration of the seizure. We all let our minds wander when we are bored, and the difference between a mild absence seizure and a fit of absentmindedness may be imperceptible, not only to the untrained observer, but to the patient himself. An absence fit lasting only a second or two may, in retrospect, seem to the patient to have been no more than a brief mental withdrawal, a quick dip in a sea of narrowed conciousness; longer seizures will have a more conspicuous effect on the patient's behaviour. He may suffer a brief loss of co-ordination. An object held in his hand may be dropped. He may stumble. His eyeballs may roll upwards, his head nod forwards, his jaw sag open. Afterwards, he may be momentarily confused, perhaps unable to recall what was happening or what was being said in the seconds immediately preceeding the fit (retrograde amnesia). More prolonged absences can develop into tonic-clonic convulsions.

Atypical absence seizures, or *absence variants* as they are sometimes known, resemble typical ones, but in addition have some focal element in them. For example, patients may have a myoclonic twitching at the side of the mouth, or in a finger or a limb, or they may utter some stereotyped phrase during a fit, which, like a typical absence, will start abruptly and last only for a matter of seconds. Some patients fall or slide to the ground and are then able to stand up immediately afterwards in what is known as an *atonic* seizure or *drop attack*. Longer seizures, where loss of muscular control may last ten to sixty seconds, followed by a period of drowsiness and stupor, are called *akinetic* seizures (akinetic means literally 'no movement').

It is not, however, by their symptoms that typical and atypical absences are most easily distinguishable from each other, but by their EEG rhythms. This is a subject that will be discussed in more detail in Chapter 4. At this stage it is sufficent to mention that the EEG rhythm, or 'brain wave', found in patients with typical absences has a monotonous and quite unmistakable uniformity, whereas the EEG rhythms characteristic of atypical absences differ according to the part of the brain in which the epileptic focus is situated.

About 40 per cent of all absence seizures occur among children, mainly before the age of ten. A quarter of all children with absence seizures will cease to have them by the age of fifteen; half will cease to have them by the age of twenty; and by the age of thirty, three-quarters will have recovered spontaneously. Of the remainder, the majority will continue to have absence seizures for the rest of their lives and about half of these will develop tonic-clonic fits. Because absences are so brief, it is not unusual for a patient to have up to 100 a day. This need not, in itself, be harmful, although too great a frequency of seizures can make it difficult for a child to concentrate and may interfere with his schoolwork.

Focal Seizures

Focal or partial seizures can be thought of as being either *simple* or *complex*. The usefulness of this distinction becomes clear if we cast our minds back to the previous chapter and recall what was said about the relationship between the brain and behaviour. Certain forms of behaviour are controlled from specific centres in the brain, such as the motor and sensory cortices, while other forms of behaviour, like thinking and memory, are the product of the integrative activity of a large number of separate parts. A simple partial seizure, therefore, is one that begins as a seizure discharge in a localized brain centre and results either in a muscular convulsion affecting one side of the body, or in some form of crude hallucinatory experience, but does not lead to any change in consciousness. Complex partial seizures are seizures that involve thought or memory or emotion, often with the addition of focal motor convulsions. Consciousness is altered, though not lost altogether; there is some dampening down, some narrowing of awareness not unlike that which occurs in a trance. The patient has, as W. G. Lennox has put it, not a black-out, but a brown-out.

Simple partial seizures

Motor Seizures: These can develop in two ways. Firstly, the seizure discharge, arising at some point in the motor cortex, can travel along the surface of the forebrain sparking off the neurons that control the different muscle groups. This does not happen in a random fashion. The seizure discharge spreads or marches along well-defined pathways. Thus, a fit that begins at the side of the mouth will march downwards into the neck and arm; a fit that begins in the fingers will march up the arm and down the legs; and a fit that begins in the feet will march up the legs and down the arms. Not every seizure will necessarily travel so far. A fit that begins in the thumb, for example, may only be followed by spasms in the fingers of the same hand. All the fits will take place on only one side of the body. Should they extend any further, then the seizure will become generalized and consciousness will be lost. This particular kind of unilateral fit (i.e. involving only half of the body) was studied in the nineteenth century by one of the greatest of English neurologists, John Hughlings Jackson, and is often known as a *Jacksonian* seizure.

Secondly, a seizure discharge may radiate out from its site of origin in such a way that certain groups of muscles go into a tonic convulsion, and the patient's body is twisted or turned in the direction of the strongest spasm. For example, the head may be turned one way and the body another. This is known as an *adversive* seizure. The direction of the twist is often away from the discharging neurons, so that a seizure discharge in the right hemisphere will produce contractions on the left-hand side of the body; and vice versa.

Sensory Seizures: The type of sensory seizure experienced by patients depends on the sense organs affected by the seizure discharge. There is a great deal of individual variation, with symptoms ranging from a vague tingling in the fingers to elaborate and precise impressions of shape, sound or smell. The point at which such seizures cease to be simple and become complex is not easy to determine, for even simple sensations — the raw data of our experience — usually have a dash of memory and emotion mixed in with them. Some of the more commonly reported symptoms include:

Vision — whirling, flashing, wavering lights; spots, stars, clouds; geometrical figures such as triangles and circles; explosions of colour — red and blue being the commonest; objects appearing larger or smaller, or nearer or more distant, or more vivid than usual. Some patients suffer from temporary blindness.

Auditory — rushing, buzzing, humming sounds in one or both ears; changes of key or pitch; sounds heard louder or softer than usual, or distorted; sounds selectively heard.

Gustatory and *olfactory* (taste and smell) — strong oppressive, pungent, bitter, sweet, sour tastes and smells. Of all sensations these are the most difficult to describe precisely. One patient compared the taste he felt during a seizure to that of a cherry; another said it was between sour and bitter; and a third said that what he experienced had the same relation to taste as tingling in the nose to smell, or a pain in the eye to vision.

Body sensations — tingling in the fingers, nausea, shivering, palpitations, sweating, blood rushing to the head. A patient's perception of his own body, its size and shape, may alter during a seizure, and he may feel larger or smaller than usual, or certain parts of his body may appear swollen. One of the most often reported symptoms consists of a feeling of discomfort or constriction in the stomach, or occasionally in the lower rectum. This is called an *epigastric* sensation.

Whenever a sensory seizure occurs prior to a generalized fit it is known as an aura. The word, which is Greek for 'breeze', was first used in an ancient medical treatise to describe the epigastric sensations experienced by a young boy with epilepsy.

Complex Partial Seizures

Complex partial seizures are sometimes also called *psychic* seizures — *psyche* being the Greek word for 'mind'. There is usually some simple motor or sensory symptoms involved as well, and the use of the joint terms *psychomotor* fit and *psychosensory* fit is meant to acknowledge this. Because many psychomotor fits are caused by lesions in the temporal lobe, there is a tendency to think that psychomotor epilepsy and temporal lobe epilepsy are the same thing. Even some doctors use the two terms interchangeably. In fact, only about half of all patients with injuries to the temporal lobes have psychomotor seizures, and only about a fifth of all patients with psychomotor seizures have lesions in the temporal lobes.

Simple motor or sensory seizures take on a new significance when memory and emotion are involved. A sound such as a rushing in the ears may form itself into a word, into a phrase, and raw shapes and colours may evolve into vivid hallucinations which, because they are caused by the action of a seizure discharge, the patient cannot help but experience. The more common symptoms include:

Hallucinations — sensations of taste and smell; hearing sounds and seeing images which do not exist except in the patient's mind. Any of the senses may be implicated, although curiously there are very few examples of patients hallucinating touch — of interpreting a tingling in the fingers, for example, as a jet of cold water on the hands. Figures seen in visual hallucinations often have a shadowy, ghost-like, sinister appearance. An hallucination is not necessarily the same as a delusion. Patients may be perfectly aware that what they are seeing only exists in their mind, but they cannot, for all that, avoid the hallucination by an act of will.

Feeling states — sudden attacks of anxiety leading to panic, often accompanied by nausea and giddiness and by epigastric sensations which appear to move up towards the throat as the seizure develops. Many patients often feel that a terrible, nameless threat is hanging over them; others have a sense of impending death. Pleasurable seizures are virtually unknown.

Distortions of memory — a feeling (by no means unique to those with epilepsy) that one's present experiences have happened before. This is called a *déjà vu* sensation, and it often takes the form of a sudden sense of familiarity, of recognition. The reverse situation, in which the familiar world suddenly and unexpectedly appears strange is known as a *jamais vu* sensation.

Dreamy states — these resemble certain forms of mental illness in which the patient is unsure about his own identity and feels unreal, fragmented, a condition called *depersonalization*; or he has the impression that the world is unreal, that life is a dream, a condition called *derealization*.

Obsessional ideas — patients feel compelled to think about a word or an idea, no matter how trivial or meaningless. Sometimes, it may be the thought of their own death they cannot avoid dwelling on. Alternatively, they may have the impression that their mind has speeded up and that they are making all kinds of extraordinary connections between apparently disparate ideas, though in fact what they are thinking may be gibberish. This is called a *flight of ideas.*

Automatisms — there are some kinds of behaviour which, although they require conscious effort to learn, can, after much practice, be carried out in a semi-automatic way; and there are other kinds of behaviour which are so complex that they demand our full attention to perform properly, no matter how many times we have done them before. For example, when we are writing we do not need to think about how to shape the letters — we learnt to do that as children; but we still need to think about what words to use. The dampening down of consciousness that occurs during a complex partial seizure makes it impossible for a patient to carry out deliberate acts, but leaves unimpaired the ability to perform those acts that are normally done semi-automatically — *automatisms* in other words. Thus, some patients smack their lips or make chewing movements during a seizure, or walk around in a drunken fashion, or break into a run, or start to undress; others utter some stereotyped phrase such as (to quote two actual examples) 'Look at the swords' or 'Come on, brother, hold these horses'. Such phrases may not always be as meaningless as they sound. One patient always repeated the words 'Forty tons of fallout' during a fit. It was only later that the doctor discovered that this was a line from a poem which, presumably, had some private significance for the patient. There are many instances of people carrying out quite elaborate acts while in a state of automatism, including driving for long distances. Jackson had a patient, a doctor, who correctly diagnosed a case of pneumonia while having a seizure. More often, though, automatic acts are recognizable by their lack of purpose. Patients may fumble with their handkerchieves or search through their handbags. During a fit, one woman loaded her washing machine with dirty dishes, another lifted up her dress in front of a stranger and a third, working in a sweet factory, stuffed chocolates into her mouth.

Complex partial seizures bear little resemblence to the popular idea of an epileptic fit and can sometimes be misdiagnosed as a form of mental illness. This is a serious mistake to make, since the drugs which are used to treat schizophrenia and severe depression tend to provoke convulsions in people with low seizure thresholds.

Status Epilepticus Seizures

An epileptic seizure is normally self-limiting: it begins spontaneously, lasts for a predictable length of time, and then comes to an end. Usually there is nothing anyone witnessing a fit need do except to keep the patient out of harm's way and to wait for nature to take its course. There are some seizures, however, which, no sooner have they ended, than they begin again, with little or no period of recovery in between, and continue until such time as the mechanisms in the brain that govern the length of a fit have reasserted themselves, or until the fit is stopped artificially by the administration of powerful sedatives, or until exhaustion and death intervene. These continuous seizures, known as *status epilepticus* fits, can be either generalized or partial. About 90 per cent of cases occur among young children, where fits lasting as long as four days have been recorded.

The most life-threatening variety of seizure is the *generalized tonic-clonic status* seizure. The body temperature, which always shoots up during a fit, can reach alarming heights if the seizures do not abate. After a while, the kidneys, lungs and heart cease to function properly and the brain becomes starved of oxygen. Among children, thirty minutes of continuous seizures can be enough to cause pemanent brain damage. Adults tend to be more resilient and are sometimes able to survive unharmed a fit lasting up to six hours. Most generalized status seizures among people with epilepsy are caused by the sudden withdrawal of anticonvulsant therapy. In patients with no previous history of epilepsy status seizures are invariably a sign of brain damage.

Absence status attacks affect mainly children and can last for hours or even days, during which time the patient appears drowsy, blinks repeatedly and can sometimes be led around.

Simple partial seizures sometimes last for many hours without becoming generalized. Usually, they take the form of myoclonic jerking in one part of the body, such as the index finger or the thumb of one hand. This form of status seizure is also known as *epilepsia partialis continua,* or *Kozhevnikov's syndrome,* after a nineteenth-century Russian physician.

About 80 per cent of automatisms last less than five minutes, but longer seizures, running into hours or even days, occasionally take place, and are known as *fugues.* Probably not all fugues are epileptic. Some would appear to be the result of various forms of sleep disorder; others are a sign of mental illness. But it is not always easy to distinguish between the different possible causes from the symptoms alone.

Status epilepticus seizures may be preceded over a period of days by an increased number of single fits, followed by recovery in the usual way. Although these *serial* fits, as they are called, may not necessarily amount to anything, they should always be viewed with concern as a possible prelude to an epileptic attack.

TABLE 1 TYPES OF EPILEPTIC SEIZURE

Generalized Seizures
A. Generalized convulsive seizures:
1. Tonic-clonic (grand mal, major)
2. Tonic
3. Clonic & myoclonic:
   (a) Infantile spasms (West's syndrome)
   (b) Lennox-Gastaut syndrome
   (c) Familial myoclonic epilepsy
B. Generalized non-convulsive seizures:
1. Typical absences (petit mal, minor)
2. Atypical absences (absence variants):
   (a) Atonic (Drop attacks)
   (b) Akinetic

Focal (Partial) Seizures
A. With simple symptoms:
1. Motor:
   (a) Tonic (adversive)
   (b) Clonic (Jacksonian)
2. Sensory:
   (a) Visual
   (b) Auditory (hearing)
   (c) Gustatory (taste)
   (d) Olfactory (smell)
   (e) Body Sensations (epigastric etc.)
B. With complex symptoms:
1. Hallucinations
2. Feeling States (anxiety, panic, nausea etc.)
3. Distortions of memory (déjà vu, jamais vu)
4. Dreamy states (depersonalization, derealization)
5. Obsessional ideas (including flights of ideas)
6. Automatisms

Status Epilepticus Seizures
A. Tonic-clonic
B. Absence
C. Simple partial (epilepsia partialis continua)
D. Complex partial (fugues)

3.

THE CAUSES OF EPILEPSY

Sometimes it is possible to say why a patient has seizures; often it is not. About two-thirds of all cases of epilepsy have no known cause and are usually presumed to be due to an inherited predisposition towards fits. Of the rest, most are attributable to infections, head injuries and tumours. The majority of cases of unknown origin (*idiopathic* epilepsy) appear before the age of twenty; while most cases of known origin (*symptomatic* epilepsy) begin in adulthood.

It can be very unsatisfactory for patients to learn that their seizures have no known cause. The need for explanation is strong in each one of us; and the most difficult facts to come to terms with are those which seem to have no reason or logic behind them. Because science is ignorant of the cause of a disease, however, does not mean it cannot provide a treatment, or even a cure. On the contrary, all diseases in history have been treated long before their causes have been fully understood.

Epilepsy is a symptom, not a disease. It is the result not of a single cause, but of the coming together — the collaboration — of many separate causes, none of which, taken by themselves, might necessarily be sufficient to provoke a seizure. The distinguished American neurologist, the late William Gordon Lennox, compared the position to that of a reservoir fed by a number of streams. At the bottom of a reservoir is an already present volume of water that represents the individual's predisposition to seizures; the height of this water is a measure of his seizure threshold. The streams flowing into the reservoir represent the various contributory causes, such as infections and tumours; and periodic overflow of the banks represents a seizure. There are, therefore, many variables at work: the water in the reservoir can be higher or lower, the streams which flow into it can be mere trickles or rushing torrents. And the likelihood of flooding can be reduced by raising the banks of the reservoir — the equivalent of taking anticonvulsant drugs.

It is often difficult to disentangle the separate causes and reduce them to some kind of order but, as a rough generalization, we can say that there are three types of causes. First, there are those which predispose a person towards epilepsy. Genetic influences, head injuries, and tumours all come into this category. There is no certainty that any of these causes will result in epilepsy; all we can say is that they often do.

Second, there are those causes which precipitate (trigger off) seizures in someone already predisposed to them. *Predisposing* causes help explain why a patient has epilepsy, but not why a fit should take place at one time and not another. The timing of individual fits is to some extent determined by the presence or absence of suitable *precipitating* causes.

The third type of cause is the most basic of all. Every epileptic seizure is ultimately due to certain biochemical factors which, by directly influencing the activity of the neurons, provoke them into behaving in an unsuitable fashion. The *biochemical* causes of epilepsy have been much researched, but are still relatively little understood.

Predisposing causes

Heredity
One person out of every 200 has epilepsy; in other words there is a 0.5 per cent chance of anyone in the community developing seizures. Where a parent has, or at some time has had, epilepsy, the chance of one of his children also having it is 2-6 per cent — four to twelve times above averge. Should both parents have epilepsy, the chances of one of their children having it rises considerably, perhaps to as high as 25 per cent, a one-in-four chance. There is thus a strong hereditary element involved in many cases of epilepsy. In what form is this passed on from one generation to the next?

With the exception of a rare form of myoclonic epilepsy, there is not any particular type of epilepsy that is inherited. There is no gene (see glossary, page 118) that transmits tonic-clonic or Jacksonian seizures from parent to child in the way that there are genes responsible for determining the colour of our eyes and hair. What is transmitted is either a low seizure threshold, which makes the individual abnormally vulnerable to seizure activity, or a disease, one of whose symptoms is epilepsy. The diseases in question are relatively rare, and it is the transmission of a low seizure threshold which is, in statistical terms, the most important factor in the inheritance of epilepsy.

Someone who is born with a low seizure threshold is more likely to have fits than someone whose seizure threshold is normal. But the mere fact that a person has a predisposition to seizure-activity does not mean that he will develop epilepsy. For this to happen all sorts of other factors must come into play. The individual may, at some time in his life, suffer a lesion to the brain that is sufficiently widespread to push him over the convulsion threshold, whereas someone else, with an identical lesion, who has no inherited tendency towards fits, may not develop them. If the appropriate precipitating cause does not come along, a person born with a low seizure threshold may go all his life without having a single fit: the streams feeding the reservoir may be so shallow that the water never rises high enough to flood the banks.

A genetic predisposition towards seizures reveals itself in EEG recordings in the form of a spike-and-wave pattern, with three spikes appearing regularly every second (see page 55). Thirty-seven per cent of the offspring of parents with epilepsy display this characteristic wave form — a much higher percentage than for the population as a whole; however, only about 25 per cent actually develop epilepsy.

An important factor to bear in mind when looking at the statistics is that not all types of epilepsy are equally likely to be inherited. If a patient acquires epilepsy as a result of a head injury sustained in car crash, it does not follow that his children will also have fits: after all, car crashes are not transmitted in our genes. Fits of symptomatic origin are, therefore, much less likely to be inherited than are idiopathic fits; and since most idiopathic fits begin in childhood, and most symptomatic fits begin in adulthood, we can say that, as a rule, the older a patient is when he first develops epilepsy, the less risk there is that his children will also have seizures.

Although the incidence of epilepsy is greater among the relations of epileptics than it is among the relations of non-epileptics, not all members of a family are equally vulnerable to the transmission of a low seizure threshold. Studies of twins have shown that, when one twin has epilepsy, the chances of the other twin also having it are far greater when the twins are identical than when they are unlike. Identical twins are, of course, much closer genetically than are unlike twins. Similarly, if the only person in your family who has seizures is an aunt or a cousin, you are less likely to develop epilepsy than you would be if it was your mother or father who was subject to seizures.

Some of the diseases that result in epilepsy are transmitted in the form of a dominant gene, which means that there is a one-in-two chance of a parent with the disease passing it on to one of his children. Into this category come *tuberous sclerosis* (epiloia) and *neurofibromatosis* (von Recklinghausen's disease). Both of these diseases are caused by a genetic disorder in the glia cells and are characterized by rashes on the body, seizures and mental retardation. *Phenylketonuria* is a disease transmitted by a recessive gene. Patients are born lacking an enzyme vital for the manufacture of protein. This, in turn, affects the functioning of the nervous system and often leads to the development of seizures. Providing it is diagnosed early enough, phenylketonuria can now be cured by feeding the child on a special diet. Two other recessive defects associated with epilepsy are the *Tay-Sachs Disease* and *Gaucher's Disease*. Both are caused by the body's failure to break down certain kinds of fats, which then accumulate in the nervous system, and result in the development of fits and mental retardation, and in premature death.

Intrauterine disorders

These are disorders which affect the child while still in the womb. They are not hereditary, but are contracted through the mother's blood supply or through the invasion of foreign organisms. *Erythroblastosis foetalis* is a disease that occurs when the foetus inherits a blood group from its father that is incompatible with that of its mother. Antibodies in the mother's blood react against the cells in the foetal blood as they would against any foreign invader, by attacking and destroying them. Many babies thus affected are born dead, and those that survive often suffer from clonic seizures and jaundice and have a short life-expectancy. Milder cases can be saved by replacing the foetal blood with a type compatible with that of the mother.

Sometimes, during its sojourn in the womb, the blood vessels in the face of the foetus become tumorous, a condition known as an *angioma*. As a result, the arterial blood is pumped too quickly round the brain, groups of neurons perish from lack of oxygen and an epileptic focus is formed. The *Sturge-Weber syndrome* is a type of foetal angioma especially associated with epilepsy.

Several types of micro-organisms, including the syphilis bacterium *Treponema pallidum*, the rubella (German measles) virus, and the parasite *Toxoplasma gondii*, can penetrate the wall of the womb and enter the foetal nervous system. The mother may miscarry, or the child may be born severely mentally retarded and prone to seizures.

Birth injuries

The greatest danger a child faces during labour, as it moves from the security of the womb to the outside world, is that at some stage it will be deprived of oxygen. *Anoxia,* or oxygen-deprivation, can occur in several ways. The umbilical cord can become wrapped round the child's throat, causing strangulation; the placenta can separate prematurely; the foetal heart-rate can drop during contractions; and the baby's head and some of the blood vessels underneath can become compressed if the mother's birth passage is narrow.

Infections

The reddening and swelling we call inflammation represents the body's normal response to the presence of an infectious agent. Inflammation of the brain is known as *encephalitis.* Between the brain and the skull are three layers of protective tissue called the *meninges.* Inflammation of the meninges is known as *meningitis.* Encephalitis can sometimes be difficult to diagnose, but the symptoms of meningitis — intense headache, fever, neck strains and a dislike of light (photophobia) — are more easily recognized.

The commonest infectious agents are viruses, bacteria and worms (helminths). A virus is a minute parasitical organism that thrives by absorbing the genetic material of the cells it attacks. Viral meningitis is not a serious condition, although when it occurs there is always a danger that the virus might spread into the brain. Some viruses are slow-acting and years may pass before their presence begins to have any noticable effect on the nervous system. Measles, which is normally a mild illness, is caused by a virus that sometimes lingers in the body after the initial symptoms have disappeared, only to re-erupt at a later date, producing a serious convulsive disorder known as *sub-acute sclerosing pan-encephalitis.* The *Jakob-Creutzfeld Syndrome* is a rare form of viral infection that results in degeneration and shrinkage of the neurons, loss of mental powers (dementia) and seizures.

Bacteria are larger than viruses, although still invisible to the naked eye. In some respects, they resemble a cross between a plant and an animal. Many cases of meningitis, especially among children, are due to bacterial infections that begin in the middle ear or the frontal sinuses. Before the discovery of streptomycin in 1944, tuberculosis, which is caused by the tubercle bacillus, was a common disease, especially among the poor. Tuberculosis can lead to seizures if the bacteria migrate from the lungs and penetrate the brain. The use of antibiotics has also reduced the number of cases of epilepsy resulting from syphillis and from blood-poisoning (septicaemia).

Worms, either in an adult form or as eggs, can enter the body through the skin, or in drinking water or on food, or they can be picked up by domestic animals from infected excreta or an infected carcass and transmitted to human beings by close physical contact. Infection by worms is more common in tropical countries than it is in Europe or the USA. The early years of this century witnessed a serious epidemic of convulsions among native troops of the Indian army caused by the pork tapeworm, *Taenia solium*. Schistosomiasis, endemic in Africa, is the result of infection by the eggs of three species of flatworm. One of these three, *Schistosoma japonicum,* can produce cysts in the brain that sometimes reach the size of an orange. Those affected often have Jacksonian seizures. In this country, the worms that parasitize sheep *(Echinococcus granulosus)* and dogs *(Toxocara canis)* are occasionally implicated in cases of epilepsy.

Trauma

Each year over a quarter of a million people in Britain receive some form of head injury. Of these, approximately 100,000 are admitted into hospital, about 5 per cent die from their injuries, and about the same number develop epilepsy. The typical victim of a head injury is a man aged between twenty and fifty. Among the people most at risk are combatants in war, motorists and their passengers, workers on building sites and at heavy engineering plants, and sportsmen, especially those who play 'contact' sports such as rugby and boxing.

The more serious a head injury, the more likely it is that a patient will develop seizures. In severe cases, the seizures may begin within a few minutes of the injury taking place. More often a week or so will pass before the patient has his first seizure. Over 50 per cent of fits occur within the first year. Probably in many cases the injury has served merely to exacerbate an already low seizure threshold. For reasons which are far from clear, however, there is sometimes a long interval between the original injury and the onset of epilepsy. One patient, an ex-policeman, who was shot in the head while trying to arrest a criminal, did not develop seizures until forty-one years later. That the gunshot wound was the cause of the fits was established when a skull X-ray revealed the presence of a small piece of shrapnel in the front of the brain. By way of explanation, it has been suggested that an epileptic focus needs time to 'mature', but there is no hard evidence for this.

There are two kinds of head injury: *penetrating wounds*, where an object, such as a fragment of a bullet, pierces the skull and embeds itself in the meninges or in the brain: and *closed wounds*, where the skull remains intact. The former kind are more often seen during wartime: a study conducted among a large group of Second World War veterans, who had suffered shrapnel wounds in the head, revealed that over a third (41.6 per cent) had developed epilepsy within three years of receiving their injury. Professor Bryan Jennett, an acknowledged authority on the subject, has stated that the chance of developing seizures from a penetrating wound is about 50 per cent. Simple fractures, on the other hand, where the meninges are not damaged, produce seizures in only about 3 per cent of cases.

Closed wounds tend to be less serious than penetrating ones, but they are not without their dangers. Sometimes a fragment of bone is pushed inwards, through the meninges to the brain, when the skull is broken. The result — a depressed fracture — is technically a closed wound, but its consequences may be the same as for a penetrating one. Even when the skull is not damaged, a severe blow to the head can still cause tearing of the blood vessels around the meninges. The blood then leaks out, forms into a clotted mass called a *haemotoma,* and puts pressure on the brain. It does not take much of a blow to the head to render a person unconscious, and where coma lasts for up to twenty-four hours there is a strong possibility of epilepsy developing. Patients may still be confused once they have regained consciousness. Amnesia is common after head injuries and the longer it continues, the greater are the chances of a patient having epilepsy.

Tumours

The cells in our body are constantly dying and being replaced, a process that normally occurs in an orderly fashion. Occasionally, though, some cells start multiplying too quickly, and if nothing is done to check their growth a mass of tissue called a *tumour* eventually forms. Tumours may remain confined to one site, such as the lungs, or they may break up and be carried through the bloodstream to other parts of the body, where they then form secondary growths.

Neurons are not altogether like other cells. We acquire our full stock of them by the end of the first year of our lives, and thereafter no more are created. Neurons lack the ability to reproduce themselves; hence, they cannot become cancerous. What is popularly called 'cancer of the brain' is the result of an excessive growth of glia cells (a *glioma*) or of the cells in the meninges (a *meningioma*).

Gliomas and healthy neurons are often so intermixed that it is sometimes impossible to remove the former without destroying the latter, but slow-growing gliomas can partially be treated over a period of time by cutting out the more accessible parts and by repeatedly draining any abcesses that form. Meningiomas, on the other hand, tend to have clearer boundaries. They can usually be successfully removed, rarely recur and are only a problem when situated within a blood vessel.

The skull, being a rigid structure, cannot accommodate any growth within it. Severe headaches resulting from the pressure of the tumour against the brain are often the first indication of the presence of a growth. At least one-third of all tumours result in epilepsy, the majority of cases being caused by slow-growing tumours. They are the commonest cause of epilepsy in people over the age of fifty.

Degenerative disorders

These are disorders which are associated with the process of ageing, although there is nothing inevitable about them. Some degenerative disorders, such as sub-acute sclerosing pan-encephalitis, are the result of infections contracted many years previously. Others may involve some genetic element which only becomes manifest in the later years of life. This is possibly the case with *Alzheimer's disease* (pre-senile dementia) in which there is a gradual loss of neurons, leading to seizures and to a deterioration in memory and behaviour.

Far more common than any of these diseases are those caused by failures in the normal functioning of the circulatory system from heart attacks and strokes.

Now that syphilis is no longer as widespread as it used to be, the most frequent cause of strokes is *arteriosclerosis*. This is due to a build-up of fatty deposits within the arterial walls. After a while, the walls become brittle and narrow and less able to respond to sudden changes in blood-pressure. A rupture (an aneurysm) forms at the weakest point, compressing the neighbouring organs and interfering with their normal functioning. Eventually, the aneurysm may burst and blood leak out (haemorrhage) into the brain. In the process neurons will be destroyed and an epileptic focus may be established. Strokes can also result from the blockage of an artery by a clot of blood (a thrombus), or by foreign matter brought from other parts of the body (an embolism).

Precipitating Causes

Given that certain people are, for a variety of reasons, predisposed towards seizure-activity, it is in most circumstances still impossible to say why a fit should take place at one time and not another. The best we can do is to describe some of the background conditions which are known to be favourable for the development of fits.

Mood

When informed (wrongly) of his wife's adultery, Othello reacts by falling into a fit. This is not just poetic licence on Shakespeare's part. Fear, anxiety, depression, or sudden rage, may all precipitate a seizure, as too may the minor, but for some people distressing, procedures of dental treatment and ear syringeing. At least one-fifth of patients with complex partial seizures attribute emotional significance to their fits. Sometimes, however, the unease that besets many patients before the start of a fit, rather than being its cause, may simply be the result of the same restless brain state that eventually gives birth to the seizure discharge.

Attention

In his book *Science and Seizures*,* Lennox observed that 'Enemy epilepsy prefers to attack when the patient is off guard, sleeping or resting or idling.' Mental activity is one of the most powerful antagonists of seizures.

*W. G. Lennox, *Science and Seizures* (Harper Bros., 1946), p.134.

Earlier it was noted that many people who would not normally be regarded as having epilepsy experience bouts of nocturnal myoclonus. Everyone, without exception, has a lower seizure threshold during sleep, when the brain's capacity to inhibit responses is reduced. And what is true of sleep is also true, and for the same reason, of those periods of inattention we all have when we are bored or fatigued. Absence seizures in particular are prone to occur at such times. The electrical impulses from the brain, the so-called brain waves, assume a very irregular shape when we are alert and become more strongly rhythmical when we relax. Such rhythmical, strongly pulsing brain waves are also characteristic of typical absences. During moments of inattention, the brain waves of the relaxed state fall into step with, and thereby enhance, the epileptic brain waves, encouraging a seizure to develop.

The subject of brain waves and their relevance to epilepsy will be discussed in more detail in Chapter 4.

Sleep

Some 44 per cent of people with epilepsy only have fits during sleep; some 33 per cent only have them when awake; and the remaining 23 per cent have them at no fixed time of the day or night. The majority of these random epilepsies are symptomatic in origin, as too are about 10 per cent of waking epilepsies. Nocturnal epilepsies are predominantly idiopathic. Seizure patterns can be remarkably regular (a fact recognised by the UK Parliament when it passed the Road Traffic Act, see page 94). It is, however, impossible to say that someone with nocturnal epilepsy will never have a fit other than at night, or that someone with waking epilepsy will never have a fit other than during the day. Seizure patterns, no matter how well-established, can sometimes change.

On first falling asleep, we go through a phase known as *quiet* or *orthodox* sleep. The muscles relax and the heartbeat, respiration rate and brain waves all slow down. Every ninety minutes or so this phase abruptly ends and is replaced by *active* sleep. We become more restless, our eyelids flicker and our brain waves quicken. In some respects we seem to sleeping more lightly, yet in fact it is more difficult to wake a person at this stage than it is during the quiet phase, an anomaly that has led some scientists to refer to the active phase as *paradoxical* sleep. Another name for it is *rapid eye movement,* or REM, sleep.

Research suggests that for people with generalized epilepsy, fits are more likely to occur during the quiet phase, when the brain waves become more rhythmical, than during the more turbulent active phase. Many patients with nocturnal epilepsy have seizures within minutes of first falling asleep. Focal seizures can erupt at any time during the night, though the EEG waves characteristic of such fits are more apparent during active sleep.

People with waking epilepsy tend to dream more during sleep than do people with nocturnal epilepsy. Since most of our dreaming takes place during the active phase, it has been suggested that, for people with nocturnal epilepsy, convulsions in some sense serve as a compensation or a substitute for lack of normal active sleep. Experiments have shown that when subjects are allowed to sleep after being deprived of active sleep for several days, they spend an unusually long time in the active phase as though making up for the deficiency. Similar experiments on animals have produced the same results; however, animals artificially made to convulse before being allowed to sleep display no excessive need for active sleep. It is still not yet clear what influence sleep patterns have on seizure activity, although it is difficult to believe there is no connection between the two. Nathaniel Kleitman has suggested that regular alternations of quiet and active phases during sleep continue to operate during the day in the form of a rest-activity cycle. If such a cycle does indeed exist it could play as important a role in determining the occurrence of seizures during the day as the quiet-active sleep cycle does at night.

Menstruation

The menstrual cycle consists of three phases covering an average of twenty-eight days. In the first (the follicular) phase, the female egg, or ovum, ripens into a kind of shell, called the Graafian follicle, under the influence of the hormone oestrogren. In the second (the luteal) phase, the ovum is released into one of the two Fallopian tubes. The follicle which is left behind grows into a small gland, the corpus luteum, that secretes the hormone progesterone. Progesterone then stimulates the lining of the womb in order to prepare it for the arrival of the fertilized egg. Should fertilization fail to occur, the corpus luteum withers and the raw surface left behind begins to bleed. This is called menstruation and represents the third and final phase of the cycle. If the ovum is fertilized, however, then menstruation does not take place and a 'missed period' is usually the first sign a woman has that she is pregnant.

One effect of oestrogen is to increase the amount of water retained in the body. Many women feel bloated and distended during the first phase of menstruation, when the flow of oestrogen is at its greatest, and sometimes put on several pounds in weight. Now, it is known that excess amounts of fluid in the tissues (hydration) can cause fits, and this may be one reason why seizures are more likely to occur during the luteal phase than at any other time in the menstrual cycle.

Oestrogen also has convulsive properties in its own right. Progesterone, on the other hand, has a sedative, slightly anti-convulsant effect on the nervous system, so that the risk of seizures is lowest immediately prior to menstruation and up to about the seventh day of the cycle, when progesterone levels are at their highest.

Drugs

Some drugs — strychnine is an obvious example — have such convulsive properties that anyone taking them, even in small amounts, will have a seizure. Epileptics are, in this respect, no different from other people. Where they have to be especially careful is in taking those drugs which normally only produce seizures in people with a low convulsive threshold. In this category come some of the more common antidepressants, particularly those that belong to the tricyclic group — including amitryptiline (e.g. Tryptizol, Saroten, Domical), nortryptyline (e.g. Aventyl, Allegron) and maprotiline (Ludiomil) — and to the MAO (monamine oxidase) inhibitors, such as phenelzine (Nardil) and mebanazine (Actomol).Among the drugs used in the treatment of schizophrenia, the phenothiazines, of which chlorpromazine (Largactil) is the most well known, also have convulsive properties.

The most widely-used drug in the Western world is alcohol. Alcohol is a sedative. It slows down the body's processes and, therefore, should — in theory — have a mildly anticonvulsant effect. According to one American survey, 79 per cent of people with epilepsy claimed never to have had a seizure after drinking alcohol; only 5 per cent said that drinking alcohol 'frequently' caused them to have fits. On the other hand, seizures are common among people who regularly consume *large* quantities of alcohol. 25 per cent of alcoholic men and 10 per cent of alcoholic women over the age of twenty-five have generalized seizures, with the peak incidence occurring between the ages of forty-five and fifty.

Some 'rum fits' are probably caused by the effects of excess fluid in the tissues. About one in ten alcoholics develop fits after head injuries following a fall. Others have seizures from forgetting to take their anticonvulsant tablets.

Alcoholism is a form of drug addiction. Not only is the alcoholic psychologically dependent on drink, but he is physically dependent on it as well. His body has adapted itself to the regular intake of alcohol to such an extent that it is no longer able to function properly without it. Significantly, many seizures take place, not during drinking bouts, but some twelve to forty-eight hours afterwards, as a form of withdrawal symptom.

Reflex Epilepsy

Some people have seizures in response to specific stimuli, such as a flickering light, a loud sound or an unexpected touch. The stimulus may grow less specific over a period of time. One man, whose fits were provoked by the sound of church music, later developed them whenever he entered, or even thought about, a church.

By far the commonest type of reflex epilepsy is *photosensitive,* or *photogenic,* epilepsy, in which seizures are triggered off by flickering lights. Driving past trees with the sunlight flashing between the branches, staring at the reflection of sunlight on water, at rotating helicopter blades, at spinning wheels — all these have been known to cause fits, while some children deliberately induce fits in themselves by waving their outspread fingers in front of their eyes.

In the early 1950s the first cases began to appear of children who developed seizures while watching defective, brightly-flickering television sets. Since then it has been found that some children have fits in front of normal-functioning sets if they sit too close to the screen, so that the picture fills the whole of their field of vision. The early onset of *television* epilepsy — most patients are aged between six and twelve years — suggests it may be partly genetic in origin. It is known that about one in twenty people with epilepsy are sensitive to the effects of flickering light. The 'flicker effect' can be simulated in the laboratory using a special kind of light known as a stroboscope that flashes on and off at a rapid pace and at a regular frequency. In the presence of a 'strobe lamp' flashing ten to twenty times a second, many patients, particularly those subject to absences, develop seizures, and even many non-epileptics are overcome by aura-like feelings of depersonalization. Flicker effects cause fits only over a limited range of frequency. The strobe lights used at discos have a relatively slow rate of flicker, and have only been responsible for a small number of reflex seizures. W. Grey Walter, one of the pioneers in the study of flicker effects, tells the story of a man who had absences whenever he cycled on fine evenings past an avenue of trees. The light flashing and sparkling between the branches induced a seizure; whereupon, he would stop pedalling. As the bike slowed down, so too did the rate at which the light flickered and his fit would come to an end.

Certain visual patterns provoke seizures in some people. One eleven-year-old girl had a fit everytime she stared at horizontal lines on a piece of material; vertical lines did not affect her. In *reading* epilepsy, it is the pattern of the letters, not the meaning of the words, that is the cause of the seizures. The way the eyes move over the pattern is also important, as in the case of the young Jewish-American boy who had an epileptic attack whenever he read Hebrew — which is written from right to left — but not when he read English. Some patients have seizures at the sight of a chess board or when looking at mathematical figures.

Reflex epilepsy can be induced through any of the senses. In *audiogenic* epilepsy, fits are caused by a specific sound, such as the ringing of bells or the whistling of a kettle. *Musicogenic* epilepsy is a type of audiogenic epilepsy in which the stimulus is a piece of music, or the sound of a particular instrument. Beethoven's Fifth Symphony and Tchaikovsky's *Waltz of the Flowers* have both been responsible for provoking fits. Some seizures occur in response to a sudden, unexpected stimulus (a *startle* stimulus), such as a loud explosion or a bright flash of light; and some in response to a light touch on the body. One elderly man had a myoclonic fit everytime his arms, shoulders or neck were touched, although a touch lower down his body had little effect on him (*tactile* or *contact* epilepsy). A few patients have fits upon making a sudden movement (*kinesigenic* epilepsy), or as a result of uncontrollable laughter (*gelastic* epilepsy).

Although it is customary to speak of reflex epilepsy as if it were a single condition, it is clear, from the variety of fits that are caused by stimuli, that they cannot all have the same origin. Photogenic seizures are usually tonic-clonic in form and primary generalized. The emotional elements in audiogenic epilepsy, the fact that it is only certain pieces of music that result in fits, suggests the presence of temporal lobe lesions. Startle stimuli usually produce myoclonic seizures that may then become secondary generalized.

Biochemical Factors

Neurons can only function properly within certain fixed limits; even slight variations in their environment can have a deleterious effect on them. Indeed, the sort of causes we have been considering up to now, such as tumours and blows to the head, as well as alterations in mood and attention, lead to the development of seizures precisely because they result in changes taking place to the chemical make-up of the neuron that lower its threshold and make it, as it were, more trigger-happy.

Oxygen and carbon dioxide

The neuron does not possess the means to store oxygen and it cannot survive without it for more than about five minutes. Oxygen is carried to the brain, and to the other parts of the body, in the red blood cells; thus, any interference in the blood supply to the brain, even for a short time, results in anoxia. Neurons die, glia cells multiply to form scar tissue and an epileptic focus is created.

The level of carbon dioxide (or, strictly speaking, carbonic acid) in the blood is monitored by a part of the brainstem known as the *medulla*. If carbon dioxide levels are high, the medulla stimulates the lungs so that we respire more quickly. As stale air is breathed out, a vacuum is created in the lungs, which fresh air rushes in to fill. Breathing, in other words, consists not so much of *inhaling* air as of *exhaling* carbon dioxide. By taking short, rapid breaths, a process known as *hyperventilation* or *overbreathing*, it is possible deliberately to override the action of the medulla and to blow off large quantities of carbon dioxide from the blood without allowing the lungs fully to reinflate. The brain becomes starved of oxygen and within a short time we feel faint and dizzy. Among people with epilepsy, especially those with absences, hyperventilation can induce a seizure in as little as ten seconds. The reasons for this are not fully understood. The effect of anoxia on neurons with a low seizure threshold is no doubt partly responsible for what happens, but there are probably other reasons as well. It is known that the neuron functions most efficiently when the fluid that surrounds it is slightly acidic. Removing carbonic acid from the blood results in the extracellular fluid becoming more alkaline, and this, in its turn, hinders the action of an important inhibitory neurotransmitter and facilitates the development of a seizure discharge.

Glucose

Glucose is a form of simple sugar produced from the breakdown of food and stored in the tissues as fuel for the body. It is 'burnt up' in contact with oxygen to produce energy. Neurons cannot store glucose any more than they can oxygen, but they can manage to exist without fresh supplies for about ninety minutes — the average length of a diabetic coma. Low blood sugar (hypoglycaemia) is sometimes a cause of fits, especially among premature babies and among diabetics who have taken an overdose of insulin. Levels of glucose in the blood are closely monitored by the brain and small amounts are released from the tissues whenever needed. Contrary to popular belief, going without a meal does not produce hypoglycaemia; extra amounts of glucose are simply made available from the body fat to make up for the deficiency.

Calcium

Calcium, which is stored in the bones, plays an important role in stabilizing the neuron and preventing overexcitation. Fits due to insufficient levels of calcium (hypocalcaemia) sometimes affect children fed on artificial milk — especially evaporated milk — high in phosphates. They do not usually occur among children who are breast-fed.

Vitamins

There is a well-established link between lack of vitamin B_6 (pyridoxine) and seizure-activity. This vitamin plays an important role in synthesizing certain neurotransmitters that exercise a restraining influence on the nervous system. In 1952, an epidemic of convulsions occurred among new-born children who had been fed on artificial milk accidentally manufactured short of pyridoxine. When the children were given the vitamin, their fits cleared up. A balanced diet provides all the vitamin B_6 required by the body, and taking extra amounts, in the form of vitamin tablets, will do nothing to improve seizure-control.

Temperature

Even a small rise in body temperature can play havoc with the delicate chemical processes that take place in the neuron. Children are especially vulnerable in this respect. Teething troubles, tonsilitis, measles and other common childhood ailments often result in a marked increase in body temperature. About 3 per cent of children with fevers develop *febrile convulsions* — as fever-induced fits are called. Viral infections are probably the commonest cause, although some genetic element may also be involved. According to one study, when one identical twin has febrile convulsions there is an 80 per cent chance of the other twin being similarly affected. Among unlike twins the risk is only about 25 per cent.

A seizure is defined as a febrile convulsion when the patient's temperature (as measured in the rectum) is at least 38°C. The fits are usually tonic-clonic, with loss of consciousness lasting fifteen minutes or less. Febrile convulsions mainly affect children between the ages of six months and five years, the majority of cases appearing between nine and twenty months.

Children are much more sensitive to the effects of anoxia than are adults. An adult brain requires about 15 per cent of the body's blood supply in order to function properly; children require about 65 per cent. A rise in body temperature of 1°C in a young child leads to a fifteen fold increase in the body's energy demands. During a febrile convulsion there is always a danger of the child's brain becoming starved of oxygen and of permanent damage being caused. The temporal lobes are especially vulnerable to anoxia and children who suffer prolonged febrile convulsions can develop complex partial seizures later in life, occasionally accompanied by some degree of paralysis down one side of the body. Happily, most cases of febrile convulsions are not serious, the patients becoming seizure-free as soon as their temperature has returned to normal. Only about one in ten of those affected will go on to develop epilepsy.

4.

THE EEG

The electrical signals emitted by groups of neurons near the surface of the brain can be detected through the skull using electrodes attached to the scalp. A record of these signals, the way they grow and lessen, become more or less frequent, or disappear altogether over a period of time, is known as an *electroencephalogram* (EEG), or brain wave tracing. There are many different kinds of EEG waves and scientists have learnt a great deal about the brain from analysing them. Electro-encephalography also has important clinical applications, especially in the field of epilepsy.

The EEG Machine

The EEG machine is a device for detecting and recording brain rhythms. It consists basically of three parts: the electrodes that pick up the brain signals; the amplifier that boosts them to a level where they can be recorded; and the write-out system that records them.

Electrodes are small discs, about the size of a shirt button, made of silver or platinum — materials that have good powers of conduction. For an EEG recording, the electrodes are arranged over the top of the head in pairs and each pair is connected to a wire that carries the signals from the brain to an amplifier, where they are magnified about a million times. On top of the EEG machine is a flat bench. A long strip of paper is driven across this bench at a constant speed by an electric motor. Suspended above the paper is a row of pens, each of which is linked through an amplifier to a pair of electrodes on the scalp. Every impulse from below the electrodes diverts a pen either upwards or downwards across the moving paper. A typical EEG machine will have about eight pens, all working independently of one another.

At the end of the recording session, the strip of paper will be covered by a pattern of jagged lines. Together these make up a graph representing the way in which the strength and duration of the brain waves have fluctuated over a measured period of time. An EEG provides only a small sample of the continuous activity of the brain; but, just as it is possible to test the purity of a river by drinking a cupful of water, so legitimate inferences about brain activity can be made on the evidence of an EEG recording lasting only fifteen minutes.

The Origins of the EEG

The science of electroencephalography dates from 1875, when the Liverpool-born physiologist, Richard Caton, first described how he had detected a flow of feeble currents in 'varying directions' — EEG waves, in other words — by placing an electrode against the exposed brains of rabbits and monkeys. His discovery was largely ignored by the scientific establishment of the day and the existence of brain waves was not fully recognized until after they had been rediscovered by two scientists working independently of each other.

Caton was also the first person to observe that brain waves, feeble though they were, could nevertheless be recorded through the skull using electrodes placed on the scalp, though neither he nor his immediate successors in the field seemed to have recognized the importance to medicine of this discovery. For a while, experiments in electroencephalography were only performed on animals whose skulls had first been opened up. Then, on 6 July 1924, the Austrian psychiatrist, Johannes (Hans) Berger made the first EEG recording on a patient using scalp electrodes. The results were encouraging and Berger continued his experiments, often using his teenage son Klaus as his subject.

Berger finally published the results of his work in 1929. Like Caton before him, his work was neglected at first, and it was only in 1934, when his experiments were successfully repeated by two Cambridge scientists, Adrian and Matthews, that Berger began to receive the recognition due to him. In the late 1930s EEG recordings were used by a team of neurologists in Boston, Massachusetts (one of whose members was W. G. Lennox) to demonstrate that psychomotor seizures were actually a form of epilespy: Jackson had suggested as much sixty years before, but it had never been proved until then. The EEG has been regularly used in the study of epilepsy ever since.

The Active and the Passive Brain

In the conscious adult, one type of EEG rhythm appears when the eyes are open and another when they are shut. Perhaps the obvious way of accounting for this difference is to say that the rhythms are produced by the presence or absence of light falling on the eyes. This was the explanation Caton offered and it was left to Berger to discover the real reason — that the two rhythms correspond to two different brain states. The one, Berger called it the passive state, occurs when we are drowsy; the other, the active state, when we are alert.

We can all recognize from our own experience the difference between the two states. Travelling to work everyday on the same bus, past the same shops and offices, in the company of the same people, we tend to ignore our surroundings. They are too familiar for us to pay them much attention and we soon lapse into a state of reverie. Should the bus suddenly screech to a halt, however, then we become instantly alert. In doing so we are merely reacting in the same way as any animal would in the presence of a novel — and potentially threatening — stimulus. We are on our guard, ready to act instantly should we need to, to fight or to flee. And so we remain until such time that we are sure we are no longer in any danger. Changes in our level of attention need not always involve such extreme situations. Every piece of new information we receive requires an attentive response if it is to be properly assimilated.

Shutting the eyes encourages relaxation by cutting out distracting visual impressions, but it is possible even with the eyes shut to produce an active brain state in subjects by asking them to pay attention to some thought or idea, or by unexpectedly ringing a bell in their hearing.

The brain rhythms that appear during the passive state Berger called the *alpha wave,* after the first letter in the Greek alphabet. As soon as the subject becomes alert and the active state takes over from the passive one, the alpha wave disappears and is replaced by a second rhythm, which Berger called the *beta wave.*

The alpha and beta waves are the two basic EEG rhythms of the conscious adult brain.

The Normal EEG

The alpha wave occurs simultaneously over both cerebral hemispheres, being strongest towards the back of the head. It is, to use the jargon, a bilaterally synchronous rhythm. The electricity emitted from the brain, like all electricity, travels in the form of waves. The distance between the peaks of the waves is known as the wavelength and the number of waves in a second as the frequency. Frequency is measured in cycles per second, or c.p.s. for short. The alpha wave has a frequency of between 8 and 13 c.p.s.; thus each single wave is between one-eighth and one-thirteenth of a second long. The synchronous nature of the alpha wave had led some scientists to describe it as a 'pacemaker' rhythm, a pulsing, metronome-like beat round which the other brain waves dance and weave.

The beta wave has a more irregular pattern. In most people,

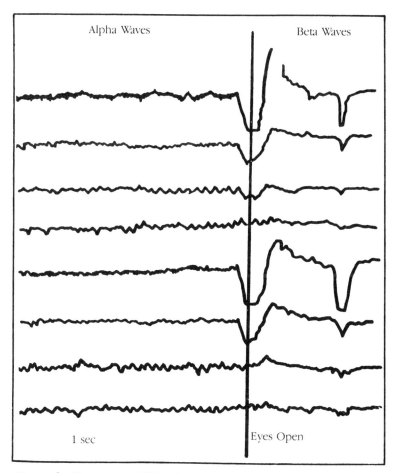

Figure 6 The normal EEG of a conscious adult. (Notice the change in rhythm from alpha to beta waves when the eyes are opened.)

it is strongest over the left — the dominant — hemisphere, particularly in the region of the frontal lobes, and it has a frequency of 13 c.p.s. and above.

As relaxation passes into drowsiness, the EEG waves become increasingly longer and slower, interspersed at first with low voltage fast activity. Theta waves, with a frequency of 4 to 7 c.p.s. begin to appear, succeeded in deep sleep by delta waves (½ to 3 c.p.s.). During sleep, the brain rhythms follow a regular sequence, with beta waves reappearing every ninety minutes or so, at the start of the active phase.

Both the theta and delta waves are a normal feature of the sleeping adult brain and of the conscious brain of the child, but their appearance in the conscious adult brain is always a sign of disease or injury.

The EEG in Epilepsy

A routine EEG examination lasts around fifteen minutes. At the end of this time, a write-out consisting of some thirty yards of paper folded into ninety pages will have been produced. Computers are sometimes used to pick out the essential features in a record, but in most cases doctors will do the interpretation for themselves. What do they look for when investigating a suspected case of epilepsy?

The EEG sign most commonly associated with epilepsy is the *spike*, a sudden, apparently spontaneous, explosion of high voltage activity that occurs against a background of normal rhythms, like a burst of static in the middle of a radio programme. A spike lasts between 20 and 200 milliseconds (msecs.), although by convention any spike longer than about 70 msecs. is known, because of its flatter shape, as a *sharp wave*. Some spikes occur in isolation; others in rhythmical sequence; and yet others are followed, as a kind of counter-reaction, by a *slow wave*, while slow waves themselves may also occur alone, especially around the site of a lesion. Another tell-tale sign is the absence of alpha or beta waves in areas of the brain where they would normally be expected.

Distortions of the normal rhythms need not necessarily be a sign of epilepsy. Certain drugs, such as phenobarbitone, generate especially fast rhythms. There is, however, one EEG feature that is consistently found in connection with one type of epileptic seizure, and this is the 3 per second spike-and-wave that occurs in cases of typical absences. As its name implies, the 3 per second spike-and-wave has a very regular pattern, with three evenly-spaced spikes erupting every second. During the seizure itself, the wave may vary slightly in frequency, but between seizures it is remarkably uniform, so much so that it is nearly always possible to diagnose the presence of typical absences from the EEG alone. Typical absences are primary generalized in origin, and there is strong evidence that the 3 per second spike-and-wave is inheritable: it is, in effect, the visible manifestation of an inbuilt low-seizure threshold. Atypical absences, which often involve some form of motor convulsion, are slightly slower (1½ to 2½ c.p.s.) and are always localized, whereas in typical absences the spike-and-wave pattern occurs simultaneously over both hemispheres.

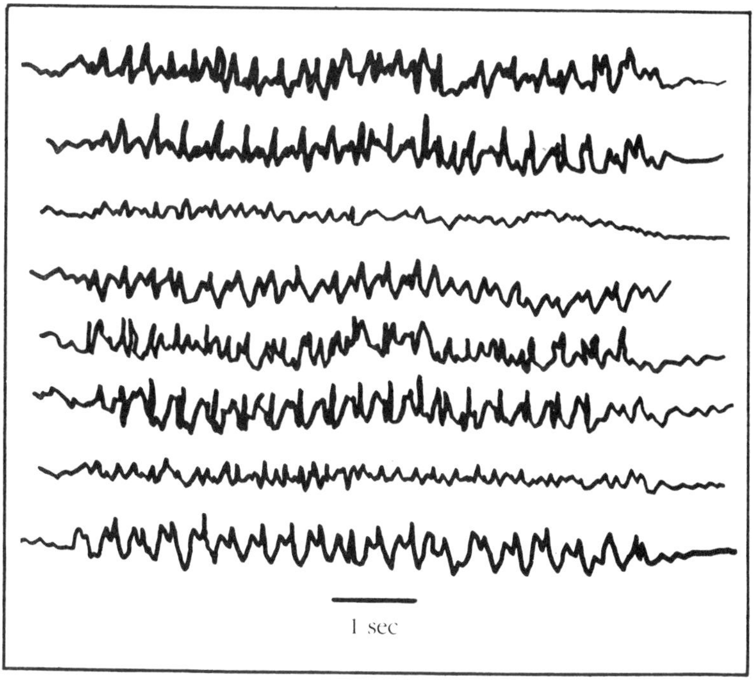

1 sec

Figure 7 The EEG of a typical absence seizure. (Note the regular, symmetrical 3 per second spike-and-wave.

The EEGs of about 60 per cent of patients with tonic-clonic seizures also show generalized but irregular bursts of 3 per second spike-and-waves, often lasting for a second or two. Where the seizures are secondary generalized, some sign of focal spiking and of slow wave activity is usually present. In the days preceding a major fit there is often an increase in the frequency of the beta rhythms; at the same time many patients report feeling increasingly anxious and uncomfortable, almost as though there was a head of steam building up inside them for which the fit, when it finally takes place, provides the explosive release. The EEG changes during the run-up to a seizure are not in themselves the cause of the patient's restlessness, but are a sign of the same

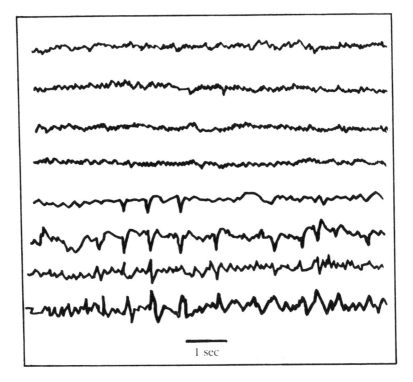

1 sec

Figure 8 The EEG of a patient with focal epilepsy. (The top four channels, recorded from the right cerebral hemisphere, display the normal alpha rhythm. But both spikes and slow waves, suggestive of some focal lesion, are displayed in the bottom four channels, recorded from the left cerebral hemisphere.)

underlying agitation in the nervous system.

During a tonic-clonic seizure, the muscles convulse so violently that it is impossible to record the patient's EEG using conventional techniques. Electrodes implanted in the brain, however, reveal that the tonic state of a grand mal fit is associated with an irregular flow of sharp and slow waves, while during the clonic stage the spikes alternate with intervals first of electrical silence and then of slow waves which swell out and become more ample as the fit comes to an end. This slow wave activity may persist against a background of normal rhythms for up to forty-eight hours after the fit, although the patient will not be aware of it.

Focal seizures are generally associated with a variety of spike and slow wave forms arising from around areas of localized injury,

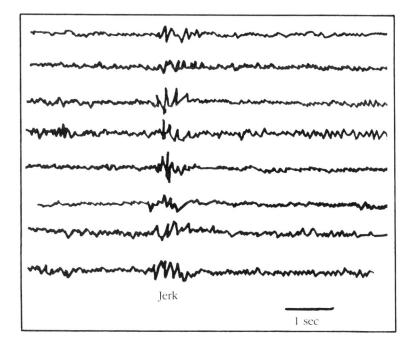

Jerk

1 sec

Figure 9 The EEG of a patient with myoclonic epilepsy. (A burst of multiple spikes and loosely associated slow waves accompany a myoclonic jerk.)

but there is often no precise correlation between an EEG abnormality and a particular type of seizure. A myoclonic jerk, for example, can sometimes occur without any corresponding change in the EEG, or a sudden spike can flare up unaccompanied by any myoclonic jerk. Also, although it is broadly the case that the motor cortex is laid out like a piano keyboard, when we look at it in more detail we find some very unexpected features, with EEG disturbances appearing over areas that control the hands or arms when a convulsion is taking place only in the leg.

Temporal lobe epilepsy shows many of the EEG signs we would expect to find in connection with any focal seizure. Above the site of the lesion itself there is a clear pattern of spikes, though

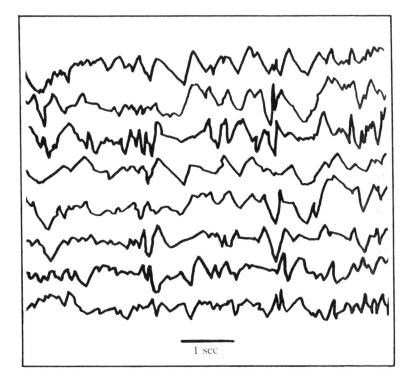

1 sec

Figure 10   The EEG of a child with infantile spasms. (Note the chaotic EEG rhythm consisting of high-voltage slow waves and random spikes.)

these tend to disappear during a seizure and to be replaced by low voltage fast activity, the waves gradually slowing down as the fit progresses. Although a patient's psychic seizures depend on the area in the brain in which the focus is situated, it is impossible to predict anything of the content of such seizures from the EEG record.

The EEG of children is more chaotic and more difficult to interpret than that of adults. Not until about the fourth year of life does the alpha wave make its appearance and another seven or eight years may pass before it begins to assume its adult form. Until then delta and theta waves predominate. In cases of febrile convulsions this chaos is quite marked, with very high voltage slow waves and spikes appearing in such a random fashion that it is often impossible to tell, just by looking at the EEG, whether a child is having a succession of fits or one prolonged fit, or whether or not he is in a coma.

The Limitations of the EEG
Berger's vision, that one day a study of brain rhythms would provide us with a fingerprint of the mind, is still far from being realized. We cannot tell anything of a person's thoughts and little of his mood by examining his EEG; and although some scientists have claimed that intelligence is directly related to the variety of the beta rhythms, there would generally seem to be no reliable difference in the EEG of a dull, but otherwise normal human being and that of an Einstein. At best all that the EEG gives us is a sketchy picture of brain activity.

There are several reasons for this imprecision, some of them more technical than others. Scalp electrodes can only detect the electrical activity of the neurons near the surface of the brain. To investigate deeper structures a more elaborate procedure, involving the implantation of electrodes, is required. Normally, twenty-two scalp electrodes are used, set about five to six centimetres apart. By placing the electrodes only two centimetres from one another, an entirely different reading may be produced. Even the speed at which the paper moves over the bench is important in determining the accuracy of the record, for the faster the paper moves, the more bunched-up and less clearly defined will be the outlines of the waves. Small but significant details may thus be blurred-out altogether.

When it comes to the study of epilepsy, electo-encephalographers are hampered by the fact that, with the exception of the 3 per second spike-and-wave, there is no single type of EEG rhythm unique to epilepsy. About 20 per cent of people with epilepsy show no EEG abnormalities, while such abnormalities can be detected in about 10 per cent of people who do not have fits. The EEG cannot normally be used to make diagnoses, but it has an important role to play in confirming them, and it is on this basis that people with epilepsy are given an EEG examination as a matter of routine.

TABLE 2 MAIN EEG RHYTHMS

Type	Frequency (c.p.s.)	Remarks
Beta	14 and higher	Normal EEG waves of alert adult brain. Asynchronous. Strongest over front of left cerebral hemisphere.
Alpha	8-13	Normal EEG wave of drowsy adult brain. Bilaterally synchronous. Strongest over rear of head.
Theta	4-7	Normal EEG wave in drowsy adult and in childhood brain. Sign of organic damage in alert adult.
Delta	½-3	Normal EEG wave in sleeping adult and in childhood brain. Sign of organic damage in alert adult.

5.

DIAGNOSIS

A doctor's immediate concern, on being called out to examine someone who has just had a fit, is to make sure that the patient has not injured himself and is recovering normally. If there is any possibility of a second fit occurring within an hour or two of the first, the doctor will administer an injection of diazepam (Valium), or some similar anticonvulsant, to raise the patient's seizure threshold. Naturally, the doctor will want to ask the patient or his family a few questions about the seizure, especially if it is the first one, but it is unlikely that he will attempt a thorough diagnosis of the fit, either at this stage or later, in his surgery. More probably he will arrange for the patient to have a consultation with a neurologist at the local hospital. Neurologists are doctors who specialize in treating disorders of the nervous system, such as epilepsy. They are concerned only with physical disease and should not be confused with psychiatrists or clinical psychologists, who deal with the problems of the mentally ill.

The Initial Interview
You have recently had your first fit. You are naturally anxious, perplexed. Your GP has made an appointment for you at your local hospital. You sit in out-patients, probably for longer than you expected, in the company of some obviously sick people, wondering what you might have in common with them. At last, your time comes. A nurse ushers you into an office. A consultant sits behind a desk . . ..

The first clinical interview can be a worrying event. You arrive wanting to know why you are having fits, yet half-fearing to hear some dreadful truth. And unless you have some idea of what information the neurologist will require from you, you may find yourself unprepared for his questions. You may also be unnecessarily disappointed if, at the end of the interview, he seems unwilling to make a final diagnosis and instead arranges for you to take some tests.

First Steps Towards a Diagnosis

One of the first clues the neurologist has when diagnosing a case of epilepsy is the patient's age. Certain types of epilepsy are more likely to begin at one time of life than at another. If the patient is a young child his fits are probably due either to an inherited disease or to an inherited low seizure threshold, although other possible causes, such as an infection contacted in the womb, or an injury sustained at birth, need also to be considered. Between the ages of about six months and five years, the effects of febrile convulsions must be taken into account. Fits that begin in puberty are frequently idiopathic in origin. Head injuries are the commonest cause of fits in early adulthood, while over the age of fifty the effects of tumours and of degenerative disorders become more prominent.

As with age, the patient's physical appearance can sometimes be revealing. An overweight, red-faced, breathless middle-aged man is much more likely to be the victim of a circulatory disorder than is a young woman or a child. Like a detective investigating a crime, a doctor works towards a diagnosis by excluding as many possibilities as he can. The patient's age and appearance are telling clues.

Early on in the interview, the neurologist will ask the patient to describe his seizures. He will want to know how long they normally last and whether or not they:

— occur at a particular time of day or night;
— are provoked by specific stimuli;
— are preceded by an aura (and, if so, what form the aura takes);
— affect one or both sides of the body;
— are clonic, tonic, or a mixture of the two;
— result in a complete or a partial loss of consciousness.

Naturally, a patient who loses consciousness during his seizures will not be able to describe them at first hand, but he should try and find out as much about them as he can by speaking to eye witnesses. Parents of a child with epilepsy should make a note of the main features of his fits as soon as they have happened:

relying on memory can lead to errors. It is very easy to imagine that a fit lasted longer than it did because of the strong emotions felt at the time.

Knowing the kind of fit a patient has helps the neurologist form a clearer idea of its possible cause. Many complex partial fits, for instance, are the result of injuries to one of the temporal lobes, whereas typical absences are usually genetic in origin. It is not just intellectual curiosity on the doctor's part that makes him want to pinpoint the seizure-type; there are also practical considerations involved. When it comes to treatment, different types of seizures respond best to different types of anticonvulsant drugs.

In order to round out his diagnosis, the neurologist will want to learn something of the patient's background, personality, tastes and habits and general medical history. In particular, he needs to know whether or not the patient:

— smokes, drives a car, plays sport etc.;
— has had any faints, convulsions, losses of memory, or strange feeling-states in the past:
— has had any major illnesses, or accidents;
— has, or has had, any relatives with epilepsy or related disorders.

The neurologist requires the same kind of information from parents of a child with epilepsy. Does the child have any problems with his schoolwork? How does he get on with his sisters, brothers, parents? If the child's mother is present, she will be asked to describe any difficulties that arose during pregnancy and labour.

Physical examination
At the end of an interview, patients will usually be required to strip to their underwear for a physical examination, in the course of which the neurologist will:

— feel the skull for any unusual variation in contour;
— examine the limbs for any lack of symmetry or for any blemishes suggestive of an organic disorder;
— feel the abdomen for the presence of any enlarged organs, and (if the patient is a woman) feel the breasts for any cysts or tumours;
— measure the pulse rate and blood-pressure;
— check for damage to the optic nerve by examining the eyes

with an ophthalmoscope;
— listen to the heart and lungs through a stethoscope for any unusual murmurs;
— test the grip for any muscular weakness;
— test the reflexes.

The neurologist can test the reflexes in two ways. First, by striking a rubber hammer against the patient's knee — producing, if the reflexes are normal, the well-known knee-jerk response. Secondly, by stroking the soles of the feet with the handle of the hammer. The normal response is for the big toe to flex downwards. New-born children, lacking a fully developed nervous system, normally respond by extending the big toes upwards. This is called the Babinski reflex and its presence in older children and in adults is usually a sign of brain damage.

A routine physical examination should last no more than about fifteen or twenty minutes. At the end of the interview, and taking into account all that he has learnt about the patient's fits and life history, the neurologist will be in a position to make an initial diagnosis. He may decide there is nothing wrong with the patient, or that the patient is ill but not epileptic. Where he suspects that the patient's seizures are a sign of epilepsy, but is still not sure of their cause, he will ask the patient to undergo a series of tests (see below). The neurologist will usually have some idea of what is wrong with the patient, but — wisely — he may refuse to commit himself to a diagnosis at this stage. Patients should be prepared to accept such doubts to begin with and to co-operate in further investigations, but they should never hesitate to express their anxieties or ask for further information. Indeed, if the doctor is doing his job properly, the initial interview should have an educative function, with the patient being presented with the facts about epilepsy, perhaps for the first time.

Epileptic-like Disorders
Before a neurologist can make a diagnosis of epilepsy, he must first satisfy himself that a patient's seizures are not the result of an unrelated condition with epileptic-like symptoms.

Faints (syncope)
Whenever we stand up for long periods, or suffer a sudden shock, our blood-pressure falls and the flow of blood to the brain is reduced. The neurons are temporarily deprived of oxygen and

we lose consciousness. Once we are prostrate on the ground, with our head and heart on the same level, the blood has no trouble in reaching the brain, even under a reduced pressure, and within a minute or two we recover consciousness.

Faints are more common among women than men. About one in 200 people faint at the sight of blood. Although most faints are not serious, they can sometimes be a symptom of a circulatory disorder, such as arteriosclerosis or the *Stokes-Adams syndrome* — a disease that causes a pronounced slowing down of the pulse rate. Occasionally, a fainting person may fall into a crouching position, with the head on a higher level than the heart. When this happens, the brain becomes starved of oxygen to such an extent that a convulsion develops. The fit might be mistaken for an epileptic one, although it is quite unrelated and need never recur. Normally we can feel a faint coming on: we grow cold and clammy and turn pale. These are totally different symptoms from those associated with epilepsy.

Sleep Disorders
Narcolepsy is a disease characterized by a sudden and irresistible desire to fall asleep. Attacks can occur at any time of the day or night, and in any situation. The patient becomes limp, drops to the ground and remains comatose for several minutes. EEG examinations of patients taken during narcoleptic attacks show that they pass immediately from consciousness into a state of active sleep without the normal intervening quiet phase. Many patients report having vivid dreams during their attacks. The typical narcoleptic patient is male, aged between ten and thirty years.

Associated with narcolepsy is a condition known as *cataplexy* in which the patient suddenly loses the use of his muscles following some strong emotional stimulus. Consciousness is retained. One patient, overwhelmed by a surge of triumph, had several cataplexic attacks while hitting a winning smash at table tennis.

Hysteria
Hysteria is an old-fashioned word used to describe a number of related psychiatric conditions. Hysteric patients sometimes express their anguish by feigning illness. In the nineteenth century, when the mentally ill, the neurotic and the epileptic were often shut up together in lunatic asylums, it was a common sight to see · hysteric patients throwing imitation seizures. This rarely happens

nowadays. Hysteric fits differ from epileptic seizures in several ways: they are more self-controlled, with patients often throwing out their arms to break their fall and — because they represent a desperate bid for understanding and sympathy — they usually occur only in the presence of other people. Some hysteric attacks vaguely resemble partial seizures, with patients making convulsive movements with their arms and legs, while choking and screaming in panic.

Migraine

The classic migraine attack consists of an intense headache over one side of the head, frequently accompanied by a feeling of nausea and an increased sensitivity to light. Many migraine patients also have additional epileptic-like symptoms, including auras and myoclonic jerks. Eighty years ago, the physician Sir William Gowers compared a migraine attack to the 'ripples in a pond into which a stone has been thrown',* and more recent research has shown that migraines are often accompanied by a slow, orderly nerve discharge that may take twenty minutes to pass from one hemisphere to the other. It is tempting to see a migraine attack as an epileptic seizure in slow motion, especially since the EEG records of some (though not all) people with migraine show signs of focal spiking more characteristic of epilepsy.

But although epilepsy and migraine may be cousins, there are some important differences between them. Epilepsy is a disorder of the central nervous system. This is less true of migraine. Some of its most typical symptoms, such as headaches, are the result of changes in the flow of arterial blood through the brain. Both epileptic and migraine attacks can be precipitated by emotional factors but, unlike epilepsy, migraine is also often an allergic reaction to certain foodstuffs and beverages, notably cheese, chocolate and red wine. There is, of course, no reason why a person should not be subject to both epilepsy and migraine. Indeed, there is some evidence that epileptics are more prone to migraine than most other people.

Miscellaneous disorders

Among other conditions that may resemble epilepsy are:

Ménière's Disease, which affects the organs of balance situated

---

*W. G. Gowers, *The Borderlands of Epilepsy* (J. A. Churchill, 1907).

in the middle ear. During attacks patients have an intense feeling of rotation and vertigo; they hear noises in their ears and fall to the ground. Over a period of time, they become increasingly deaf.

Breathholding attacks and hyperventilation. Found predominantly among children, breathholding attacks and hyperventilation may cause seizures but, unlike epilepsy, are often deliberately induced, perhaps as part of a temper tantrum.

Drop attacks. These differ from epileptic drop attacks in that they are not the result of a seizure discharge. Both weakness in the thigh muscles and disease in the arteries in the brainstem cause some middle-aged people to pitch forwards on their knees without losing consciousness.

Carotid sinus disorder. Towards the bottom of the carotid artery is a slight enlargement (the carotid sinus) containing nerves that monitor changes in blood-pressure. In some people, the carotid sinus is abnormally sensitive. Even slight pressure on it (such as may occur when buttoning up a shirt collar) can lead to a sudden slowing of the heart, followed by a faint.

Nervous tics. Some people, mainly children, have facial twitches that resemble myoclonic jerks. Such tics, however, do not originate from an epileptic focus, but are a sign of emotional disturbance.

Investigative Techniques
A short while after the initial interview with the neurologist has taken place, the patient will be asked to attend his local hospital in order to undergo tests. Because such tests cost money to perform, and because they are always inconvenient and sometimes distressing to the patient, only the minimum number will be carried out. Such a pragmatic approach may offend those patients who feel that no stone should be left unturned when it comes to investigating the possible causes of their seizures. In the overwhelming majority of cases, however, there is no justification for submitting patients to tests that will do nothing to improve their treatment.

The EEG examination
As we saw in the last chapter, an EEG machine is a device that detects and records the electrical activity of the brain. It does not generate electricity and there is no connection between an EEG examination and electro-therapy.

An EEG examination is an entirely painless affair. The patient remains fully conscious throughout, either sitting on a chair or lying on a couch, and no anaesthetics of any sort are used. At one time, patients used to be asked not to take their anticonvulsants during the twelve hours preceeding the examination in case the presence of the drugs in the brain masked any abnormal EEG rhythms. Now, however, it is realized that most anticonvulsants leave traces in the blood for much longer than twelve hours, and that giving them up for the examination does little to improve the quality of the results and only serves to put the patient at risk. The only exception to this is if the patient is taking a drug derived from benzodiazepine, such as diazepam (Valium) and nitrazepam (Mogadon).

Before the EEG examination can begin, the technician who carries it out must first fit the recording electrodes to the patient's scalp. There are two kinds of electrodes in daily use. One kind is struck onto the scalp using harmless glue called collodion that is then dried with a jet of air. Afterwards, a conducting jelly is squeezed through a hole in the centre of the electrode. The other, and more commonly used, kind of electrode consists of a plastic mount with a silver rod on top. At one end of the rod is a pad of cotton wool covered in lint that has previously been soaked in a saline solution. The patient dons a rubber cap that resembles a cross between a hairnet and a cyclist's crash helmet. This is then tied under the chin with a strap. Next, the electrodes are pushed between the slats in the cap and finally the wires that carry the electrical impulses from the brain to the EEG machine are fitted to the electrodes with crocodile clips. The stick-on type of electrode has a wire built into it. Grease on the hair tends to interfere with the weak electrical signals emitted through the skull and so patients should have a thorough shampoo before taking an EEG examination and avoid using a hair spray or hair oil.

The brain is not the only part of the body to emit electrical signals. So too do all the muscles, including the heart, and bursts of static electricity come from our clothes everytime we move. The room in which the EEG examination takes place is insulated to prevent interference from mains electricity, radios and other pieces of electrical equipment and the EEG machine itself is designed in such a way that most extraneous signals, or *artifacts* as they are called, are excluded from the recording. However, patients should try to keep still during the recording session, in case the electrical signals from their muscles should drown out those from the brain.

At the start of the examination, the patient is asked to open and shut his eyes several times while the technician observes the familiar alternation of the alpha and beta rhythms. The signals from the eyelids and eye muscles appear on the record as bursts of increased voltage against a background of normal rhythms. The patient is then asked to hyperventilate for two and a half to three minutes and to look at a stroboscope flashing at 1 to 60 c.p.s. Both hyperventilation and photic stimulation are effective means of releasing abnormal rhythms that otherwise might remain hidden. The technician keeps a constant eye on the print-out from the machine and should it become apparent to him, from the nature of the brain waves, that the patient is on the verge of having a fit, then he will immediately stop the examination.

Taking into account the time spent fixing and unfixing the electrodes, an EEG examination usually lasts about half an hour. This is convenient for the patient, but it does sometimes mean that the EEG record may not always be as representative of brain activity as a doctor might wish. In recent years Oxford Medical Systems have developed a miniature EEG machine in which the scalp electrodes are connected to a battery-operated cassette, weighing less than a pound (455g), that can be worn on a belt around the waist. The Medilog, as this device is known, makes it possible for a twenty-four hour EEG record to be made without imposing undue restrictions on the patient.

Lumbar puncture

A *lumbar puncture* is a relatively simple proceedure. The patient is given a local anaesthetic, then a hollow needle is inserted into his back, between two of the lumbar vertebra at the base of the spine, and a sample of cerebrospinal fluid is drawn off. Cerebrospinal fluid is a watery solution that surrounds the brain and the spinal cord. Patients with suspected meningitis are usually given a lumbar puncture and their cerebrospinal fluid is tested for any abnormalities; but the technique is not used routinely in the diagnosis of epilepsy.

Radiography

Most patients with epilepsy will have their chests and skulls X-rayed. Chest X-rays became a routine form of medical investigation in the days when tuberculosis was rife. Nowadays they are more frequently given to identify the presence of cancers. Either situation is relevant to epilepsy, for seizures can be caused both by infection with the tubercle bacteria and by tumours whose primary site is the lungs.

Although often used to reveal distortions in the shape of the skull, X-ray photography is of limited value when it comes to investigating possible lesions in the brain. No matter from which angle an X-ray photograph is taken, the different structures of the brain always appear superimposed on one another. One way round the problem is to introduce into the brain a harmless material that enhances the differences in density between different tissues. The more dense a tissue is, the more X-rays it will absorb and the whiter it will appear on the photographic negative. In *air encephalography (pneumoencephalography)*, the patient first undergoes a lumbar puncture, after which a small quantity of air is introduced into the spinal canal through a hollow needle. The air rises up the spine and fills the hollows at the centre of the brain known as the ventricles. These stand out clearly when photographed, enabling a doctor to recognize any abnormalities in their size and shape. Air encephalography is a safe but distressing form of examination. While it is taking place, the patient has the unpleasant sensation that his head is being blown up like a balloon; and it may take a couple of days for the headache to clear up.

In an *arteriogram,* a solution containing iodine is injected into one of the carotid arteries (or through a catheter in the region of the carotid arteries) while the patient is under a general anaesthetic. Iodine, like air, absorbs more X-rays than the surounding tissues, and its presence in the blood vessels of the brain serves to highlight any abnormalities that may be present.

Computed axial tomography

The fact that the brain is composed of tissues of different densities, which causes such problems in conventional X-ray photography, is turned to good advantage in the technique of *computed axial tomograghy.* A CT (CAT, or EMI) scan is an instrument that compares the amount of X-rays entering the skull with the amount leaving it. By deducting the second figure from the first, it is possible to obtain a measurement of the number of X-rays absorbed by the brain, and hence of the density of its various tissues. The patient lies on a bench with his head between two X-ray detectors. The CT scan is slowly rotated, a degree at a time, and a cross-sectional picture of the brain is built up. The information from the detectors is stored on a computer as a sequence of numbers that can be translated into a visual image for the purposes of diagnosis. Tumours, having a different density from the surrounding healthy tissue, can thus be pinpointed, no matter what part of the brain they are situated in, although additional techniques may be needed to discover the precise nature of the tumour. A CT scan uses lower doses of X-rays than conventional radiographic methods and is, therefore, much safer.

Although the original paper on computed axial tomography was written in 1961, the instruments themselves did not become widely-available until about ten years ago; yet already CT scanning looks as though it may soon be replaced by two newer techniques, *nuclear magnetic resonance* and *positron emission tomography,* which analyse the structure of the brain according to the amount of energy consumed by the different tissues.

Other tests
Patients are often asked to give specimens of urine and blood, which are then examined for signs of glucose and mineral deficiency. A microscopic analysis of a piece of the patient's tissue, removed in simple and harmless fashion from the wall of the rectum, is sometimes taken in order to confirm a diagnosis of tuberous sclerosis or neurofibromatosis. Epileptic children with developmental problems may be given a psychological examination, in which factors such as intelligence, and language and motor skills are assessed. Patients who are being considered for an operation to remove an epileptic focus may have miniature electrodes made of silver wire implanted in the brain, a technique known as *stereotactic depth encephalography.*

6.

TREATMENT

There are a number of different treatments for epilepsy available. Only surgery offers the possibility of a cure, and then only in very limited circumstances. The overwhelming majority of patients require anticonvulsant drugs to control their seizures. These drugs can be injected into a vein or a muscle, or given as a drip, but normally they are swallowed as tablets, capsules, syrups or liquids (suspensions).

How Anticonvulsant Drugs Work

Once an anticonvulsant drug has been swallowed, it passes down the gullet to the stomach; then, after being dissolved by the digestive juices, it is absorbed through the walls of the intestine into the bloodstream and is circulated round the body. Only when it reaches the brain does it begin to have an anticonvulsant effect. Quite how such drugs work is still not fully known, but it is generally supposed that they retard the more excitable neurons from discharging and thus help to raise the seizure threshold.

From the body's point of view, an anticonvulsant drug is an alien substance. Every time it passes through the liver the drug is systematically broken down into an inactive form. It is then expelled into the bladder and finally excreted in the urine. After several hours, the anticonvulsant becomes so thinly concentrated in the bloodstream as to be no longer effective and the patient must then take another dose of the drug to prevent a seizure from occurring.

The Principles of Drug Treatment

There is now a wide range of anticonvulsant drugs available. In deciding which one to prescribe to a patient, a doctor will first bear in mind that, for each type of seizure, a drug exists which laboratory research and clinical experience together indicate as the most suitable. Only if that drug proves unsatisfactory will a doctor then prescribe a drug of 'second choice', or a combination of two or more different types of drugs. When it comes to deciding how much of an anticonvulsant to administer, the doctor's aim is to reach a happy compromise: too little of the drug and it ceases to prevent seizures, too much and it produces harmful side-effects.

All other things being equal, a large, heavy person will require more of a drug than does someone who is small and light in stature. This is obvious enough, but there are complicating factors which make the prescribing of drugs a much more uncertain matter than it might at first appear. What doctors also need to bear in mind is that:

— The quicker the liver breaks down, or metabolizes, a drug, the more of that drug a patient must take to achieve the required results. Children have a higher metabolic rate than adults and therefore must be given proportionally larger doses of a drug, whereas it may be necessary to reduce the amount given to an older person, as the body's metabolism tends to slow down with increasing age.

— Some drugs are metabolized more quickly than others. Most anticonvulsants break down relatively slowly so that it is usually sufficient to take them only once or twice a day.

— The liver can metabolize some drugs efficiently only up to a certain point. Beyond that, it finds it progressively more difficult to deal with additional amounts of the same drug and quite small increases can greatly enhance the risk of harmful side-effects developing.

— After some drugs have been given for a period of time, their presence may actually stimulate the liver to metabolize at a faster rate. Dosages that were once effective no longer remain so, and it becomes necessary to give more of the drug in order to achieve the same results as before.

— It is possible to overcome the side-effects of some drugs, without reducing their efficiency, by taking them regularly. The fact that a patient may grow used to a drug he at first found hard to tolerate is not necessarily a sign that the drug is no longer working properly.

— If patients are prescribed more than one drug, the way those drugs interact will influence their individual effectiveness.

Drug Treatment in Practice

The prescribing of drugs is partly a matter of science and partly a matter of trial-and-error. It is now possible to measure with some accuracy the amount of a drug active in the body from a sample of the patient's blood. During the early days of treatment, the patient will be given a blood serum test (as it is called) at frequent intervals. If it is found that serum levels are below normal, then the doctor may feel it is worthwhile administering a slightly higher dose of the drug to a patient in order to strengthen seizure control. If, on the other hand, the level of the drug in the bloodstream is above average, then the doctor may think it wise to reduce the dosage level, or even to switch to another drug.

Measurement of serum levels provides a good guide to the way a patient's body is handling a drug, but cannot be used to predict how much of a drug a patient will need. People vary greatly in their reactions to drugs and it may take several months of trial and error to discover the anticonvulsant and the dosage level most suitable for the patient. Even once a suitable drug regime has been worked out, patients should be given a fresh blood serum test every three years or so to ensure that their response to the drug has not changed imperceptibly in the meantime. Growing children require even more frequent check-ups.

Patients have a vital role to play in the working-out of a suitable drug regime. They should not think of themselves as guinea pigs passively taking whatever is handed them. If the doctor is to do his job properly he will need to know not only whether the drugs have prevented a patient's fits from taking place, but also whether they have produced any harmful side-effects. Often, the patient is the only person in a position to know this. It is a good idea for patients to keep a diary while their drug regime is being worked out and to note down the dates of any seizures that occur and the circumstances surrounding them, as well as any side-effects they may observe.

A patient's drug regime will have been decided upon by the same hospital-based neurologist who carried out the initial interview. Should an occasion arise when the patient becomes anxious or dissatisfied about the drugs he is taking, then his first step should be to consult his local GP, who will, if he thinks it necessary, arrange for the patient to see the neurologist.

Types of anticonvulsant drugs

All drugs are known by at least two names. The company

responsible for manufacturing the drug sells it under a *proprietary,* or trade, name, unique to them. New drugs may be only manufactured by one company and, therefore, have only one proprietary name, whereas more well-established drugs may be sold under several different proprietary names. To avoid confusion, each drug is also given a *generic,* or approved, name. English-speaking countries tend to use the same generic names, but differ over the proprietary ones. Phenytoin, for example, is the generic name for an anticonvulsant drug marketed in the UK as Epanutin and in the USA, Canada, Australia and New Zealand as Dilantin. A doctor may use either type of name when writing a prescription.

Drugs Commonly Used to Treat Epilepsy

Phenytoin (Epanutin, Dilantin)

This is probably the most widely-used of all anticonvulsants. It is the drug of first choice for the treatment of generalized tonic-clonic seizures, both primary and secondary, and it is also regularly used in cases of focal epilepsy, often in combination with other drugs, notably sulthiame, carbamazepine and phenobarbitone. *Side-effects:* After it has been taken for about three months, phenytoin begins to cause excess growth of gum tissue (gingival hyperplasia). The gums become soft and spongy, bleed easily and look unsightly. The condition tends to stabilize after a while. It is possible to cut the gums back to their original level, but the procedure is painful and protracted and there is no guarantee that it will have any permanent effect. Good dental hygiene is essential to avoid the build-up of plaque. Patients should brush their teeth and gums at least twice a day and use dental floss, and they should consult a dentist or a dental hygienist at least every six months. Such measures will keep gum damage to a minimum, while a slight degree of hyperplasia might be thought a price worth paying for effective seizure-control. Phenytoin can cause excess growth of body and facial hair (especially at first), nausea, and double vision.

Carbamazepine (Tegretol)

This drug has similar pharmacological properties to phenytoin, but as it does not cause excessive hair growth it is often preferred when treating female patients. It can be used for most kinds of seizures, especially generalized tonic-clonic and focal ones, but is ineffective in cases of absence fits. It should be administered in small doses at first to avoid drowsiness and a blood serum test should be given twice a week. Later, as the patient adapts to the drug, levels can be increased and blood serum tested every one or two months. Although a relatively safe drug, carbamazepine should not be introduced to female patients during the first three months of their preganancy in order to avoid any possible risk of birth defects.

Side-effects: Allergic skin reactions, drowsiness, nausea, dry mouth. Very occasionally carbamazepine causes a disease in which there is deficiency of white cells in the blood (aplastic anaemia) and jaundice.

Ethosuximide (Zarontin)

This is the drug of first choice for the treatment of absence seizures. It is also often effective in controlling myoclonic and atonic fits, but it has no value in the treatment of generalized tonic-clonic seizures, and indeed may exacerbate them. Patients who have both absence and tonic-clonic seizures, and who are treated with ethosuximide for their absences will need to be given a second drug to control their tonic-clonic fits.

Side-effects: Skin rashes, nausea and vomiting, and drowsiness.

Sodium valproate (Epilim, Depakene)

This is the newest anticonvulsant drug, having been in regular use only since the 1960s. It has proved successful in treating most kinds of fits, including typical absences and myoclonic seizures, and appears to have very few side-effects. Tablets of Epilim easily absorb moisture and should be kept in their foil-wrapped packs until needed. Most patients will want to swallow them with water in order to avoid the burning sensation that occurs if the tablets begin to dissolve in the throat or upper intestinal tract.

Side-effects: Nausea, some weight loss (though this is only short-lived), and a tendency to bruise easily.

Phenobarbitone (Gadrenal, Luminal)

Phenobarbitone is the oldest anticonvulsant drug still in use, having been around since 1912. It is cheap and reasonably safe and, although it is now rarely used as a drug of first choice, it still has a role to play in cases of generalized epilepsy that have proved resistant to other forms of treatment. In January 1985 phenobarbitone was added (along with all other barbiturates) to the list of controlled drugs covered by the Misuse of Drugs Act 1971. Police officers have been instructed by the Home Office not to confiscate the drug from anyone requiring it for the treatment of epilepsy, but as a precaution the British Epilepsy Association advise all patients taking phenobarbitone to carry with them a BEA identity card containing a signed statement from their doctor.

*Side-effects:*Phenobarbitone is a sedative and it frequently produces drowsiness and lethargy, sometimes accompanied by unsteadiness of gait and poor co-ordination (ataxia). The psychic symptoms of temporal lobe epilepsy may be exacerbated by taking the drug. It makes some children restless and irritable and occasionally causes skin rashes.

Diazepam (Valium), nitrazepam (Mogodon) and clonazepam (Rivotril, Clonopin)

These three are included together because they all belong to the same family of drugs, the benzodiazepines. Diazepam is best-known for its use as a minor tranquillizer, nitrazepam as a 'sleeping pill'. In the field of epilepsy, diazepam and clonazepam are used mainly in the treatment of status epilepticus. Injected into the patient they quickly bring the fit to an end. Given by mouth, nitrazepam has value in the treatment of myolonic epilepsy. Diazepam is the drug of first choice for dealing with febrile convulsions.

Side-effects; Drowsiness, fatigue, ataxia. Clonazepam sometimes causes irritability and aggressiveness.

Drugs of 'Second Choice'

Methoin (Mephenytoin; Mesontoin, Mesantoin) and Ethotoin (Peganone)

These two drugs belong to the same family as phenytoin (the hydantoins). Methoin is stronger and more toxic than phenytoin, ethotoin less so. Both can be used for the treatment of generalized tonic-clonic and focal seizures. The greater sedative properties of methoin makes it a suitable drug for those cases that have proved resistant to the use of phenytoin.

Side-effects: Similar to phenytoin, except that neither drug causes excess growth of gums or hair. Methoin can produce serious liver damage if not monitored closely.

Acetazolamide (Diamox)

Acetazolamide is a drug of second choice for the treatment of absence fits and is often administered in conjunction with phenytoin or carbamazepine. Because of its diuretic properties, it is sometimes given to women whose seizures are associated with the menstrual period.

Side-effects; Nausea, headaches, fatigue, flushes.

Sulthiame (Ospolot)

This is mainly used in the treatment of partial seizures, often with phenytoin. Indeed, its anticonvulsant effects may be largely due to the fact that it causes phenytoin levels in the blood to rise.

Side-effects. Headaches, nausea, drowsiness, hyperventilation, mental confusion.

Troxidone (Tridione) and paramethadione (Paradione)

Introduced as a pain-killer in 1929, the anticonvulsant properties of troxidone were first recognized during the Second World War. Although it offered the first effective treatment for absences, troxidone has since been superseded by less toxic drugs. However, it is still occasionally used as a drug of second choice, especially when given with phenytoin. Paramethadione is pharmacologically similar to troxidone.

Side-effects: Drowsiness, sensitivity to light (photophobia) and skin rashes. Patients taking these drugs should have a serum test at least once a month to avoid the risk of bone marrow disease.

Primidone (Mysoline)

When taken, primidone is partly converted in the body to phenobarbitone. It is a useful drug of second choice for the treatment of most kinds of seizures, including primary and secondary generalized tonic-clonic and myoclonic fits.

Side-effects: Primidone can cause excessive drowsiness in anyone unused to the drug and, therefore, it must be given in lower-than-therapeutic doses at first, then increased gradually over a period of weeks until the correct level is reached. It also causes ataxia and skin rashes in some people and occasionally is responsible for a condition in which there is a deficiency in the number of red cells in the blood (megaloblastic anaemia).

Methylphenobarbitone (Prominal)

This is chemically very similar to phenobarbitone. It can be used for treating the same types of epilepsy and has the same side-effects.

Phensuximide (Milontin) and methsuximide (Celontin)
Both these drugs are similar to ethosuximide. Methsuximide is the most potent of the three. Phensuximide does not exacerbate tonic-clonic seizures in the way that ethosuximide often does, but is less effective in controlling seizures.
Side-effects: Similar to ethosuximide.

Adrenocorticotropic hormone (ACTH).
ACTH is of value in the treatment of infantile spasms, particularly when these are the result of brain damage; but it is not a drug that can be given for any length of time without causing serious and potentially fatal organic disturbances.

Other Forms of Treatment

Surgery
Surgery is an appropriate form of treatment for only relatively few people with epilepsy. If one leaves aside those cases where the patient's life is under immediate threat from a tumour or a head injury, surgery is normally only carried out on epileptics able to meet a strict set of criteria. Firstly, their epilepsy must be serious enough to warrant the considerable time, effort and expense required to perform a major surgical operation. Removing or destroying cerebral tissue is always an irreversible act, and there is no justification for putting a patient at risk unless his seizures are so bad as to make any kind of normal life impossible.

Secondly, an operation can only be undertaken when the site of the epileptic focus is known — this rules out all cases of idiopathic epilepsy — and is accessible. A surgeon may decide it is better to leave a focus in place rather than to destroy healthy tissue in trying to remove it. Gliomas are often inoperable for this reason.

Thirdly, surgery will only be attempted when every other form of treatment has proved unsuccessful: it is always a method of last resort.

Finally, surgery will never be carried out on children, for whom some chance of spontaneous recovery exists.

Before an operation can be performed, the patient must first undergo a rigorous series of tests designed to locate the precise site of the focus. Electrodes, invisible to the naked eye, will be implanted in his brain and left in place for about twenty-four hours in order to monitor local changes in EEG rhythms. He may be given a convulsive drug and a seizure will be induced to see how his brain reacts. Also he will probably receive a detailed psychological examination.

The brain does not feel pain; all its sensations are referred to other parts of the body. In the standard surgical treatment for epilepsy, developed during the 1940s by a team from the Montreal Neurological Institute led by Wilder Penfield, only a local anaesthetic is used: the patient remains conscious throughout the operation. The surgeon first cuts a section through the skull and folds back the meninges underneath; then, using an electrode to administer a series of brief electric shocks, he searches for the precise site of the focus. Each shock simulates the action of a seizure discharge; when the electrode is placed on the motor cortex, for instance, the patient's limbs automatically convulse. Most people with epilepsy who receive surgery have complex partial seizures, and their symptoms are often only obvious to themselves. Thus, as the surgeon moves the electrode from spot to spot, he asks the patient to describe what he is feeling. When at last the patient's sensations are the same as those which normally occur during one of his seizures, the surgeon knows he has at last come into contact with the epileptic focus. This can then be sucked out.

Penfield's use of electro-stimulation has played an important part in mapping out the different functional areas of the brain, but as a surgical tool it has come in for some criticism in recent years. Now, there is an increasing trend for surgical operations for epilepsy to be performed on fully anaesthetized patients, with the surgeon removing not just the focus but a whole secton of a lobe, as a single block of tissue, a procedure known as a *lobectomy*. The patient's co-operation can still be invaluable, however, when the surgeon is attempting to remove a focus situated close to an important functional area, such as one of the speech centres, which it is vital to avoid damaging.

Sometimes the surgeon will destroy a focus *in situ* by implanting radioactive seeds or by using radio-frequency currents. In rare cases, an entire hemisphere may be cut away. Some patients with severe fits have been helped by an operation in which the corpus callosum has been severed, thus preventing the spread of the seizure discharge from one hemisphere to the other. This procedure, known as a *commissurtomy,* has led to some bizarre side-effects. Without an intact corpus callosum, the nerve messages transmitted from the fingers on the left hand to the right side of the brain are no longer relayed to the speech centres in the left hemisphere, with the result that the patient finds himself at a loss to name unseen objects held in his left hand in spite of being able to identify them by touch. The patient is, in effect, possessed of two brains, neither of which is on speaking terms with the other.

Counterstimulation
It has been known for many centuries now that a focal seizure can sometimes be aborted by applying a counterstimulant to the area in convulsion. For example, a fit that begins with the forcible closure of the patient's hand may be prevented from spreading by forcing the hand open. Medieval physicians, using this same principle, are said to have arrested seizures by burning blisters on their patients' skin.

The American neurologist, I.S. Cooper, has made a scientific study of counterstimulation and applied it with some success to the treatment of epilepsy. His research has been concentrated on the cerebellum, the part of the brain responsible for fine-tuning and co-ordinating movement. Every time a nerve message is sent from the motor cortex, an identical message is despatched to the cerebellum. The cerebellum also receives sensory messages from the limbs as they move and is thus able to compare the original commands to the muscles with their actual performance. This information is then passed back to the motor cortex, where it exerts an influence over any subsequent messages that are sent. What Cooper has done is to intercept this elaborate feedback mechanism by directly stimulating the cerebellum, which then reacts as it would if the muscles were in convulsion by sending a stream of inhibitory messages to the motor cortex. The technique appears to be most effective when an electric current of approximately the same frequency as the alpha rhythm (10 c.p.s.) is used. Faster frequencies (over 200 c.p.s.) cause the inhibitory neurons in the cerebellum to become 'fatigued' and allow the seizure discharge to develop with greater rapidity than it would have done had the stimulus not been applied in the first place.

Cooper has fitted some patients with a battery-powered transmitter, worn on a belt round the waist, which can be used to stimulate the cerebellum whenever a seizure seems imminent.

Antennae taped on the chest carry a radio signal from the transmitter to a receiver, a few centimetres in diameter, situated beneath the collar bone. This in turn is connected by a wire under the skin to a set of platinum electrodes implanted in the cerebellum. In a more sophisticated version of the same device a signal is automatically transmitted to the brain in response to changes in brain waves monitored by a portable EEG machine. One patient who benefitted from Cooper's invention was an eighteen-year-old boy with a history of seizures accompanied by aggressive behaviour, including attempted suicide. When the wire from the transmitter broke one day, the boy had thirteen seizures. As soon as the machine was fixed, his condition stabilized.

Biofeedback

Biofeedback is a method of helping patients alter certain physiological functions that are normally thought of as being beyond conscious control. It has been used with some success in treating people with anxiety states and high blood-pressure.

In the early 1970s Barry Sterman of UCLA discovered that cats trained to enhance a particular brain rhythm localized to the motor and sensory cortices became seizure-resistant when exposed to noxious chemicals. Sterman's findings have been extended to the treatment of epilepsy and some patients have been taught to suppress slow rhythms associated with seizures and to induce faster ones in their place with the help of an EEG machine wired up in such a way that, whenever the chosen rhythms appear, a light flashes on. The light provides patients with the feedback, the constant flow of information, they require in order to judge their own performance. With practice, they become sensitive to the kinds of sensations that accompany the flashing of the light and eventually are able, by adopting the right frame of mind, to summon up the desired brain waves at will.

Biofeedback training has proved moderately successful with some patients, whose seizures had previously resisted any form of control, but it is a difficult and time-consuming technique to learn and constant practice is needed if satisfactory results are to be maintained.

Diet

During the 1920s there was a vogue for treating epilepsy with special diets. In the *hydration diet* patients were allowed only three glasses of fluid a day; watery foods, including fruit, were forbidden them. Since some seizures are indeed caused by an excess of liquid in the tissues, the hydration diet was not wholly unscientific, but it was of little value to the majority of people with epilepsy. Much the same can be said of the *starvation diet*, which required patients to fast for at least forty-eight hours. When the body is deprived of food, it resorts to burning up its own stores of fat and protein for energy. In the process ketone acids are released in the blood. As we noted in connection with hyperventilation, slight increases in acidity (acidosis) have an anticonvulsant effect.

It is not, however, necessary to starve a person in order to obtain acidosis. The same state can be achieved, while at the same time allowing for an adequate daily intake of calories, by eating foods low in carbohydrates and starch and high in fats. This is the basis of the *ketogenic diet*. There is nothing especially new about it. In the Middle Ages Arab physicians sometimes prescribed a diet of fat meats 'up to the point of disgust and nausea' as a remedy for epilepsy.

The ketogenic diet is still used, mainly in the treatment of young children whose seizures cannot be controlled by drugs. The expensive and unpalatable animal fats that were once the staple ingredient of the diet have been partly replaced in recent years by triglyceride oils. Strict supervision is needed if the ketogenic diet is to work properly and for this reason it is often used only on patients in hospital. Should the child be kept on this diet at home, then his parents must ensure that he does not cheat by eating other foods. Care must be taken to prepare the diet accurately and a daily urine test must be carried out to monitor its effects on the system.

TABLE 3 MAIN ANTICONVULSANT DRUGS

Generic Name	Proprietary Name	Preparation
Drugs of first choice		
Phenytoin	Epanutin, Dilantin	tablets 25, 50, 100mg capsules 50, 100mg suspension 30mg/5ml
Carbamazepine	Tegretol	tablets, 100, 200mg syrup 100mg/5ml
Ethosuximide	Zarontin	capsules 250mg syrup 250mg/5ml
Sodium valproate	Epilim, Depakene	tablets 200, 500mg syrup 200mg/5ml
Phenobarbitone	Gadrenal, Luminal	tablets 15, 30, 60mg capsules 100mg
Diazepam	Valium	tablets 2, 5, 10mg
Nitrazepam	Mogodon	tablets 5, 10mg
Clonazepam	Rivotril, Clonopin	tablets 0.5, 2mg
Drugs of second choice		
Methoin	Mesontoin, Mesantoin	tablets 100mg
Ethotoin	Peganone	tablets 250mg, 500mg.
Acetazolamide	Diamox	tablets 250mg
Sulthiame	Ospolot	tablets 50, 200mg
Troxidone	Tridione	capsules 300mg
Paramethadione	Paradione	capsules 300mg
Primidone	Mysoline	tablets 250mg
Methylphenobarbitone	Prominal	tablets 30, 60, 200mg
Phensuximide	Milontin	capsules 500mg
Methsuximide	Celontin	capsules 300mg

7.

EPILEPSY: SOME ISSUES

Sexual Relations

There is no reason why someone with epilepsy should not have sexual intercourse: only rarely does an orgasm result in a seizure. But anxiety over having fits is sometimes a cause of sexual problems. According to one study, some two-thirds of men with temporal lobe epilepsy suffer from impotence, although many of those interviewed enjoyed a satisfactory sex life before their illness. Sexual problems appear to be no more common among epileptics with other types of seizures than they are among non-epileptics.

Patients sometimes blame their anticonvulsant drugs for their loss of sex drive. Phenobarbitone and primidone are the most complained of in this respect, although it is not always clear whether it is the drugs themselves or some other, mainly psychological, factor that is responsible; however, anticonvulsants can make a person listless and apathetic if taken in excess. Some anticonvulsants, notably phenytoin, primidone, phenobarbitone and carbamazepine, interact with the contraceptive pill and, by causing it to break down quicker than normal, render it less efficient. Women using these particular anticonvulsants would be well-advised to consult their doctor or their local Family Planning Clinic and to explore other forms of contraception.

There are many myths about the relationship between sex and epilepsy. It is not true that a woman who plays the active role in the sex act, or who has sex during pregnancy, will give birth to a child with epilepsy; and it is equally untrue that fits are caused by masturbation or by over-indulgence in sex.

Having Children

Until recently legislation existed in the United Kingdom and the

USA to discourage people with epilepsy from having children. In some instances epilepsy was regarded as a bar to marriage; in others as grounds for divorce. Although anyone with epilepsy is now free to marry and to start a family, there is still often some doubt in the minds of those concerned as to the wisdom of doing so. What factors need to be considered before a rational decision can be made?

To begin with, it has to be admitted that some people whose fits are poorly controlled may find it difficult to hold down a regular job; and if there is little money coming into a household, the additional expense of caring for a child can put strain on a marriage. Women who have frequent seizures need to consider whether or not they will be healthy enough to go through with a pregnancy and to look after a young child. A husband with poor seizure-control may already be dependent on his wife to such an extent that she would have no time left over to care for a child. A woman with epilepsy may feel that she is perfectly capable of being a mother if only her husband was prepared to take an equal share in bringing up a child. This involves a wider consideration of the way husbands and wives see their respective roles in marriage — considerations which of course, are not restricted in their relevance to people with epilepsy. When the marriage (or relationship) is a genuinely co-operative one, with husband and wife sharing equally the burden of childcare, then there is probably no reason why epilepsy — of itself — need present any undue problems.

However, what of the chances of a child inheriting epilepsy from its parents? This has often been seen as the main argument against people with epilepsy having children. The statistics of heredity have already been discussed in Chapter 2. To summarize them briefly: in cases of idiopathic epilepsy, where one parent has a low seizure threshold and the other parent is seizure-free, there is a 2 to 6 per cent chance of a child inheriting a similar threshold to his epileptic parent, though it does not follow from this that he will develop fits. Where both parents have a low seizure threshold, the chances of one of their children being similarly affected increases to about 25 per cent. In the case of those neurological disorders, such as tuberous sclerosis, in which poor seizure control is but one among a number of symptoms, the risk of inheriting the disorder depends on whether it is spread by a dominant or a recessive gene, and whether one or both parents are affected, but is, broadly speaking, quite high.

Partners who are worried in case their children should have seizures should consider closely the type of seizure activity they are considering. Where a partner developed fits in adulthood, the chance of one of his children developing fits is only slightly greater than average, and in those circumstances — all other things being equal - one might confidently advise such a couple to start a family should they want to. Similarly, where only one partner has a low seizure threshold, there is still only a small possibility that one of their children will also develop epilepsy. There is, however, an increased chance of such a child having febrile convulsions during infancy, and although these may turn out to have no lasting effect, would-be parents should be aware of the risks involved and the action they should take should such an event occur.

In the majority of cases, there is no good reason why people with epilepsy should not have children. To suggest otherwise is to fall into the old trap of thinking of epileptics as helpless souls incapable of living a normal life. Whilst no one would choose to have epilepsy, I am sure that most people would prefer to be born with epilepsy than not be born at all. The idea that a parent who gives birth to an epileptic child is somehow responsible for corrupting the 'purity of the race' is an obscene one which, if we have learnt anything from recent history, ought never to be taken seriously again.

Those who want further advice on the matter should first visit their local doctor, who will be able to put them in touch with the specialist services of a genetic counselling clinic.

Pregnancy

Since a woman puts on weight during pregnancy, any anti-convulsants she is taking will be dispersed among a larger volume of tissue, and this might suggest that, unless her drug intake is stepped up, she will have more seizures when carrying a child than at other times. This is certainly the case with some women, but it is also true that other women have fewer fits during pregnancy, while others again continue to have fits at the same frequency as before. It is impossible to predict what will happen to any specific individual. A blood serum test will show whether a pregnant woman needs to take more anticonvulsants, and changes in dosage levels can be made if necessary. However, women should not increase the number of tablets they take without first seeking the advice of a doctor, nor for that matter should they stop taking them from a mistaken belief that pregnancy is a cure for epilepsy. It isn't, and a woman who suddenly stops taking her anticonvulsants puts her own life and the life of her unborn child at risk.

A pregnant woman with epilepsy should let her obstetrician know of her medical condition and should regularly attend the clinic where the levels of anticonvulsants in her blood and her general state of health can be closely monitored. Doctors prefer on the whole for women with epilepsy to have their children delivered in hospital in case any complications should arise. A dangerous convulsive disorder known as *eclampsia* can occur during the final stages of pregnancy. The cause of the condition is unknown, but it is thought to be the result of a toxic infection. It is not, however, a form of epilepsy.

Small quantities of the mother's anti-epileptic drugs will be absorbed by the foetus through the bloodstream. This is inevitable, but it need not, in most cases, cause any undue problems. Foetal abnormalities only occur in about 7 per cent of cases. Many of the children affected are born below weight or have only mild conditions, such as cleft palate, but some are more seriously ill with heart defects and bleeding problems. The off-spring of mothers using phenobarbitone, phenytoin and primidone appear to be most at risk. It has been suggested that women on these drugs should take vitamin K tablets during their last month of pregnancy and be given vitamin K in a drip during labour, but there is no general agreement on this.

A baby born to a mother taking phenobarbitone or diazepam may be excessively drowsy for the first few days after birth, but should recover once the last residues of these drugs have been excreted in its urine. If, however, the baby continues to absorb small quantities of anticonvulsants through its mother's milk, then it may remain drowsy, and in these circumstances it would be advisable for a woman to give up breast-feeding and to bottle-feed instead.

Education

The child with epilepsy has the same educative needs and the same needs for friendship and self-expression as any other child. Whenever possible, he should be educated within the normal school system. If it is necessary to make allowances for him because of his epilepsy, then these should be kept to a minimum. At the same time, it should be realized that a child's performance at school could be influenced by his having fits, especially if the teaching staff fail to recognize them when they occur and think that he is merely being lazy or inattentive. A balance must be struck. Nothing should be done to make the child feel he is freakish because he sometimes has seizures, but nor must his health be put at risk by refusing to give him the special consideration he may need on occasions.

Parents should let the child's class teacher know of his epilepsy. A private conversation, possibly accompanied by a letter from the child's doctor, will often be all that is required when dealing with a conscientious and informed teacher. What is important is that the teacher should understand the true facts about epilepsy, that he should be alert to any possible effect a child's seizures might have on his work and his relations with other pupils, and that he should know how to cope if a child has a fit at school. Teacher and parents should also be in agreement as to what — if any — restrictions should be placed on the child. Should he be allowed to swim, for instance? And if he does can the teacher ensure that skilled supervision will be given? The parents should explain in detail to the teacher the form that their child's fits assume — how long they last, how long it takes for the child to return to consciousness, and so on — so that the teacher will be in a position to know if medical aid is required should a fit occur. The British Epilepsy Association issue a number of free leaflets which explain the basic facts of epilepsy in a clear and precise way, and parents should not hesitate to provide copies of these to the child's teacher if they think it might help. Whether or not they also wish to approach the headteacher must be a matter for personal choice. Certainly, they should always do so if they are not satisfied with the class teacher's attitude towards the subject.

A child's performance at school can be adversely affected by having epilepsy in at least one of four ways;

— children who suffer from frequent seizures may have difficulty concentrating in class and remembering what they have been taught;

— children who are taking too many, or the wrong kinds of, anti-epileptic drugs may be drowsy and inattentive;

— children who have other neurological problems in addition to epilepsy may have genuine and permanent difficulties in learning and may require special teaching in order to make full use of the abilities they do have; and

— children who feel persecuted for being epileptic, or are in some way emotionally disturbed, may find school work difficult and may be very unwilling to go to school.

A teacher should be aware of these possibilities when judging the school work of a child with epilepsy. He or she should consult the parents of any child who displays some of the following symptoms in class; staring spells, or daydreaming; head drooping, eye rolling; purposeless sounds and body movements; excessive chewing and swallowing; sudden tic-like jerks of the body or head; repetitive nodding or blinking; and a general lack of response.

Children who have very frequent seizures, or who have other neurological disorders in addition to epilepsy, often benefit from being educated at a special school. There are six such schools in England, and one in Scotland, and together they accommodate about 1 per cent of the estimated 70,000 schoolchildren with epilepsy. All the schools offer the normal educational facilities as well as medical care and their staffs include teachers, doctors, nurses, physiotherapists, occupational therapists, and other ancillary workers. Application to them should be made through the local education authority.

As a matter of long-term policy, however, it is questionable whether so-called handicapped children should be educated separately. Ideally, there should be a single state system which, whilst providing for the specific medical needs of individual pupils, nevertheless allows all children to mix together, irrespective of their mental or physical capacities. Until this is done there will always be a tendency among the healthy majority to regard the handicapped as problems rather than as people.

Special Care
In Britain, patients who are prevented by their seizures from maintaining themselves, and who cannot be looked after at home, can at present be cared for at one of the centres for epilepsy, such as the David Lewis Centre in Cheshire and the Meath Home for Epileptic Women and Girls in Surrey. Known originally by the unpleasing name of colonies, these centres were mostly founded by Victorian philanthropists in order to provide residential care for long-stay patients, many of whom, although only mildly affected by seizures, had other neurological disorders as well.

At the time it was believed that people with disabilities fared best in a condition of rural solitude, segregated from the general community. Colonies were built to be self-sufficent, with their own farms, market gardens and workshops. They soon became overlarge, impersonal places. Much-needed reforms were introduced in the 1960s. Greater emphasis is now placed on rehabilitation. Standards of assessment and care have improved and closer links have been forged with university departments and special clinics. Some 2,000 people at present live in the centres for epilepsy and another 3,000 are housed in the various forms of special accommodation supported by local government.

The centres still have a role to play in providing a wide-range of specialist services, mainly for short-term patients, but increasingly the need is for the establishment of more hostels in residential areas. Hostels offer a less institutionalized way of life than the old colonies did. They put patients and their relatives within convenient travelling distance of one another, and they generally make it easier for the individual to become integrated into the community.

Employment

A recent survey of the social difficulties faced by people with epilepsy revealed that over half (54.9 per cent) of those questioned regarded 'employment' as their commonest problem. Naturally, much depends on the kind of job a person does, or wishes to do. Someone seeking an academic career will probably find that having epilepsy is not regarded by employers as a serious problem. The most disadvantaged in this respect are unskilled and semi-skilled workers. Increasing levels of unemployment make matters worse: when there are many people competing for the same job, applicants who have seizures are likely to be at a disadvantage.

Although people with epilepsy are often thought of as making unreliable workers, the evidence suggests the opposite. Studies in Great Britain and the United States have shown that someone with epilepsy is no more likely to have an accident at work, or need long periods of sick leave, than any other employee. Some employers make the excuse that their workers would object to working alongside a person who has fits, although it is doubtful if many of the employers who say this have ever consulted their workers on the matter. Prejudice against people with epilepsy does exist at work, among all grades, but refusing a job to someone for fear of stirring up that prejudice can only make it worse.

It is sometimes said that epileptics should not work with machinery in case they injure themselves during a fit. There are two points to be made here: firstly, under the Health and Safety Regulations employers have a duty to put protective guards round all the moving parts of a machine and generally to make it hard for anybody, whatever the circumstances, to injure themselves in a fall; and secondly, when people have a fit they usually fall backwards or sidewards, rather than forwards. This is not to say there might not be some danger in some people with epilepsy working with machines, but it is a danger that has been exaggerated in the past, and it has no doubt resulted in many people with epilepsy being refused work in factories which it would be safe for them to do.

Whether or not an applicant for a job reveals the fact of his epilepsy will depend to a great extent on the attitude of the employer. If he is perceived as being understanding, the applicant may well feel he can tell him the truth, although the nature of the job and the desperation of the applicant to find work will also play a part. According to a recent survey, over half of those who had had two or more full-time jobs after the onset of epilepsy had never told their employers about their condition, while one-tenth had always told them. People who conceal the truth from their employers may find themselves plagued with worry in case they are found out, and worry can sometimes bring on a fit.

An applicant who does not mention his epilepsy at a job interview, who is taken on, and who subsequently has a fit at work, risks dismissal on the grounds of breach of contract. Whether or not an industrial tribunal will uphold such a dismissal depends on several factors. If there was a question on the application form asking 'Are you subject to fits?' and the applicant answered 'No', knowing that he was, he may lose his case. Even if no such question was asked, a dismissal might be deemed fair if it was felt that the applicant's state of health was relevant to the job he was applying for. On the other hand, if there was no good reason why someone with epilepsy should not do the job in question, an industrial tribunal might decide that the employer had acted unfairly and order him to pay compensation to the dismissed worker.

People with epilepsy are forbidden to join the police, the fire brigade, the armed services and the merchant navy, to drive heavy goods vehicles and to teach physical education. There are also certain types of work which, although it is not illegal, it might sometimes be unwise for a person with epilepsy to do. These include: work on high buildings, moving vehicles or isolated sites; jobs near open water, exposed electrical circuits or unguarded fires; jobs that involve regular foreign postings or that deal with valuable, fragile equipment, or with small children. None the less, there are probably people with epilepsy in all of these jobs.

Anyone who is uncertain as to the kind of work for which he is medically suited should contact his local Job Centre who will put him in touch with the Employment Medical Advisory Service, a branch of the Health and Safety Executive. Here he will receive a free medical examination and free advice from a qualified doctor. Most Job Centres have a Disablement Resettlement Officer (DRO) on their staff, a person who specializes in finding work for people with medical conditions such as epilepsy. The DRO may suggest a course of work preparation and assessment at an Employment Rehabilitation Centre and this may lead to training at a government Skillcentre, a training college for disabled people, or a commercial college paid for by the Manpower Services Commission (who run the Job Centres). The MSC also finances a job introduction scheme to encourage employers to take on more workers. Skillcentre training is only available to skilled and semi-skilled workers and some of the more popular courses have a waiting list of up to two years.

People with epilepsy can register as disabled at their Job Centre, although it is not necessary to be registered in order to have an interview with a DRO. Since an Act passed in 1944, all firms employing over twenty people have been required to recruit at least 3 per cent of their workforce from the Disablement Register. Unfortunately, the quota system is not strictly enforced. Anyone with epilepsy who applies for a job as a registered disabled person will probably find himself in competition with other disabled people, and some employers prefer to give work only to those who have a conspicuous physical handicap.

Insurance

Life assurance premiums are calculated from figures that show the average life-expectancy of different groups of people. The extent to which these group statistics can fairly be used to estimate the premium for any single individual depends on how comprehensive they are. Insurance underwriters, who can draw on the records of large numbers of people, collected over many years, are much better placed to estimate individual differences than they would be if only a small sample was available to them. Because of the relative paucity of data about the mortality rates of people with epilepsy, there is a tendency, especially among more conservative insurance companies, to treat all patients alike, irrespective of the type of seizure they have, or the degree of their seizure-control, or their general state of health, or their age, occupation and personal circumstances. Epileptics with a normal life expectancy are thus charged punitive rates merely because they are deemed to belong to a category which includes some patients with a poor life-expectancy.

People with epilepsy who wish to take out a life assurance policy are advised to consult a specialist broker first. Tyser and Company are probably the most experienced in this field. Working closely with the British Epilepsy Association, Tysers recognize the wide differences that exist among patients and claim to be able to place the majority of the applications they receive. Policies are generally small, and some people whose earnings are limited by virtue of their epilepsy may be unable to meet the minimum premium, which (in 1986) is about £10 a month. Endowments and other policies that carry an investment content are easier to place than are Term and Whole life assurance (see glossary). The amount of excess ('loading') companies charge people with epilepsy varies from 50 to 100 per cent for Term assurance, though it is sometimes possible, if the patient remains in good health over a period of a year or two, to re-negotiate some reduction in this.

Anyone (under the age of seventy) who becomes a member of the British Epilepsy Association automatically receives a personal accident policy with benefit of up to £1,000. The BEA also offer motor insurance for members with epilepsy who are eligible to drive, and travel insurance to members with epilepsy travelling abroad. One of the objects of these insurance schemes is to provide the Association and their agents, Tyser and Company, with details of the kinds of claims made by epileptics. Improved actuarial figures will make it easier for underwriters to distinguish between the risks attaching to different individuals and to offer fairer premiums.

Motoring

People with epilepsy are permitted to drive a motor vehicle under certain circumstances. The legal position is set out in the Motor Vehicles (Driving Licences) (Amendment) (No. 3) Regulations 1982. These state that a person with epilepsy is eligible for a driving licence providing that:

— they have had no epileptic seizures during the two years immediately preceeding the application; or
— that for the last three years their seizures have occurred only during sleep; and
— that by driving a vehicle they are not likely to be a source of danger to the public.

To apply for a licence you should first obtain form D1 from your local post office. Question 6d on the form asks, 'Have you now or have you ever had epilepsy? If you answer 'Yes' to this question, then you will be sent a questionnaire and asked to give details of your medical history, the names and addresses of the doctors who have treated you, and permission for these doctors to be consulted by the Department of Transport about your case. Should the Licensing Authority's Medical Officer be satisfied with the information he receives, then he will issue you with a licence. If there is some doubt, he can ask for a second opinion, or refer your case to the Honorary Medical Advisory Panel, or do both, and the Department will bear any costs incurred should you have to undergo a medical examination.

If you object to the decision of the Licensing Authority you can appeal to the Magistrate's Court, and if you are unsatisfied with the verdict you receive, and there is a point of law at issue, you can take your case to the High Court. Since this is a civil matter, you will not be entitled to legal aid, and if you do have seizures, it is difficult to see how you can win your case.

If your application is successful, a licence will be issued to you for a period of one to three years and will be renewable free of charge providing there has been no change in your medical condition in the meantime. It is your responsiblity (not your doctor's) to inform the Department of Transport should you have a seizure after the licence has been granted and to surrender your licence to them. If you have no fits for a further two years, you can ask for your licence to be returned. Similarly, if you were issued with a licence before the onset of epilepsy, you must surrender it to the Department and let them know of your changed medical condition.

The main object of the regulations is to protect the public against injury from drivers who have a seizure at the wheel. Nocturnal epilepsy apart, no distinction is made between types of fits. The fact that your seizures only occur infrequently, or are always preceeded by an aura that gives you time to lie down before you lose consciousness, or are only of a short duration — none of this is considered relevant by the Licensing Authority, neither is the claim that, without a car you may lose your job, or be housebound. Put like this, the regulations may seem harsh; but they are not unreasonable bearing in mind the result of a survey which showed that, out of 2,500 road accidents due to medical causes, 50 per cent were attributable to epileptic activity.

Under the Heavy Goods Vehicles (Drivers' Licences) Regulations 1977 and the Heavy Goods Vehicles (Drivers' Licences) (Amendment) 1982 no one who has had a seizure since the age of five years can lawfully drive a heavy goods vehicle. Identical restrictions apply to the driving of public service vehicles (i.e. buses and coaches).

8.

SOME COMMON QUESTIONS

What Should I Do If I See Someone Having an Epileptic Seizure?

Absence Seizures
Often it is unnecessary to mention to the patient that you have observed him having a fit. If he has absences regularly, he may well take them for granted and not thank you for drawing attention to them. Offer quiet reassurance if he seems confused. *Never* react as though a major tragedy has happened. It hasn't.

Febrile convulsions
Strip off the child's clothes and sponge his body with tepid water, to help bring down the fever. If the convulsions last for more than ten minutes, call a doctor.

Simple partial seizures
Make sure there are no objects on which the patient might hurt himself should he fall down. Otherwise do nothing. *Never* try to stop a muscular convulsion by pinning down the patient's limbs. You won't succeed and you may injure yourself and him in the attempt.

Complex partial seizures
Steer the patient away from any dangerous objects, but — unless he is about to hurt himself — *don't* try to restrain him. Some patients interpret restraint as a form of aggression and become aggressive in return. *Don't* badger the patient with questions once he has recovered, or react as though you have just witnessed something extraordinary. Calm solicitude is all the patient requires, and there are limits even to that.

Generalized tonic-clonic seizures

Don't push anything into the patient's mouth to prevent him from biting his tongue. You could break his teeth. And while a bitten tongue will heal, broken teeth will not. Also, some patients vomit at the end of a fit, and if there is something stuck in their throat at the time, they could choke. *Don't* hold down the patient's limbs. Move him only if he is in danger of hurting himself. *Don't* try to give him a drink before he has fully returned to consciousness.

While the fit is taking place, put a cushion or a rolled-up jacket under the patient's head and — if possible — loosen his shirt collar, or any other article of tight clothing. *Don't* do anything else until the patient's limbs have stopped jerking and it is clear the fit is over. Then turn the patient on his side in a semi-prone position, with his knees slightly bent and his head lower than the rest of his body. Wipe away any mucous or saliva from around his mouth and check that there is nothing obstructing his breathing.

Usually patients come to no harm during their fits, but accidents do occasionally happen and it is as well to be prepared for them. If the patient's tongue rolls to the back of his throat during a fit and obstructs his breathing, then you should quickly turn him on his side in a semi-prone position. The tongue should then lie flat against the bottom of the mouth. Remember, though, that it is normal for the patient's complexion to turn blue-grey in colour during the tonic stage of the fit, so don't misinterpret this as a danger signal.

If the patient has difficulty in breathing *after* the fit has ceased, then gently slip a finger, or a spoon handle, or a pen, or some similar object, into his mouth and press his tongue down. Never thump the patient (or anyone else) on the back to remove an obstruction from the throat. The blow will make him inhale instinctively, and the obstruction will be drawn even further down the windpipe. Instead, turn the patient so that his head is pointing to the ground, get behind him, put both your arms round his waist and sharply squeeze him in the abdomen. Hopefully, the obstruction should then be dislodged as he exhales.

It will not normally be necessary to call for medical help. You should do so only:

— if the fit lasts longer than five minutes;
— if a second fit develops immediately after the first one has ended;

— if the patient does not recover consciousness within fifteen minutes of the end of the fit; or

— if he has injured himself badly. An injured patient should be kept warm, but not moved; wounds should be covered with a light, clean material and the rate of bleeding slowed down by applying gentle pressure to the affected area.

Can You Outgrow Epilepsy?

Whether people who cease after a while to have seizures can be said to have outgrown them is a moot point. We simply do not know why remission occurs. That it happens, though, and happens often, especially among patients whose seizures begin in childhood, is beyond doubt. A detailed study conducted in the USA at the famous Mayo Clinic, and covering a period of nearly forty years, came to the conclusion that, ten years after the onset of epilepsy, the chances of recovering from it were 75 per cent for those whose seizures began before the age of ten, 68 per cent for those whose seizures began between the ages of ten and nineteen, and 63 per cent for those whose seizures began between the ages of twenty and fifty-five. Twenty years after the initial diagnosis, approximately 30 per cent of patients continued to have seizures, approximately 20 per cent still took anticonvulsants, but had been free of seizures for five years, and approximately 50 per cent had been free of seizures for the same period, unaided by medication. The greatest likelihood of remission was among patients with generalized tonic-clonic epilepsy (85 per cent), followed by those with absences (80 per cent) and partial complex seizures (65 per cent). Spontaneous recovery occurred least frequently (46 per cent) among patients with other neurological problems besides epilepsy.

Other studies support the findings of the Mayo Clinic study and allow us to make certain generalizations concerning the probability of remission. We know, for example, that a patient is more likely to stop having fits if he was a child when his seizures began, if he had only a few seizures before being diagnosed, if he has idiopathic epilepsy, if he has generalized tonic-clonic fits, and if he has no additional neurological disorders. The quality of treatment a patient receives is also an important, though less easily quantifiable, factor. In the Third World, where medical standards are frequently lower than in the West, epilepsy affects at least eight people in every 1,000 compared to about five in every 1,000 in the UK.

Do Frequent Seizures Lead to Brain Damage?

Pathologists have occasionally reported finding signs of extensive cell damage in the brains of epileptic patients. These post-mortem results have been interpreted by some scientists as evidence that frequent seizures can produce permanent injuries to the brain. There are good reasons to doubt this, however. The epileptics whose brains have been studied after death have usually come from special centres and been more severely handicapped than most other people with epilepsy. One cannot safely generalize about all patients from such a limited sample. Moreover, it is often impossible to tell from microscopic examination alone whether neuronal injury is the result of frequent seizure-activity, or of some viral or degenerative disease unconnected with epilepsy. A seizure discharge, after all, is only a form of neural conduction, and the nerve cells in our brains are firing all the time without showing any signs of stress. Indeed, it would be surprising if they did, for it is the job of the neuron to fire: that is what nature has designed if for. A sustained status seizure can cause brain damage, due to anoxia, but the majority of seizures do not last long enough to be dangerous.

It has sometimes been claimed that brain damage is a slow, cumulative process, lasting over many years, and that each fit, though insignificant in itself, causes a slight degree of wear and tear, which extends and deepens with the passage of time. According to this theory, the brain is like an airplane suffering from metal fatigue that flies for thousands of miles without any problems, and then suddenly cracks up. If this were the case, then one would expect to find that the most disabled patients were those who had absence seizures, since these occur with far greater frequency than any other type of fit. But the evidence suggests otherwise. Studies by Lennox have shown that neither frequent minor, nor infrequent major seizures have any harmful effect on the majority of people with epilepsy, although frequent major seizures may. As up to 80 per cent of patients find that their fits are well-controlled by medication, the chances of epilepsy causing brain damage would seem to be very, very small indeed.

Do Seizures Affect Intelligence?

Epilepsy and mental retardation are sometimes associated. For instance, about a third of all severely subnormal children have fits. Epilepsy is not a cause of mental retardation, however, just as mental retardation is not a cause of epilepsy. Both are symptoms which often occur independently of each other, but which sometimes occur together in certain neurological disorders. The majority of these are identifiable soon after birth; a few appear later in life. The intellect of patients who do not have any of these disorders is usually unimpaired. Statistics show that up to about 80 per cent of people with epilepsy are of normal intelligence; around 20 to 30 per cent are of below normal intelligence; and about 2 per cent are of above normal intelligence — Julius Caesar and the Russian novelist Dostoevsky both had epilepsy.

Young children with epilepsy sometimes show signs of mental impairment when they are taking too many, or the wrong kind of, anticonvulsant drugs, or when their seizures are poorly-controlled. Neither situation need be irreversible. And it is often the case that children whose school performance is unexpectedly poor display a dramatic improvement once their seizures have been brought under control.

Do Seizures Affect the Personality?

At one time it was thought that people with epilepsy all had certain character traits in common such as jealousy, moodiness, inflexibility and petty-mindedness. We now know that this is not true. The theory of the 'epileptic personality' was based only on the behaviour of seriously disturbed patients, many of whom had spent years in institutions, and it was never applicable to the majority of people with epilepsy. Nevertheless, up to a third of epileptics face social difficulties of one kind or another as a result of having seizures. What are the reasons for this?

Some patients find it hard to live a normal social life because of the prejudices against epilepsy that exist. Isolation, repeated failures, and rejection can lead to withdrawal and depression. Anticonvulsant drugs provide a ready instrument for committing suicide and the numbers of epileptics who attempt to take their own life is above the average rate. Prejudice is often internalized by its victims. Epileptics who are brought up to think of seizures as a sign of inadequacy may develop strong feelings of guilt or shame. They see their epilepsy as something to be hidden, apologized for, resented. Lacking self-esteem, they make a poor impression on others and, in doing so, inadvertently confirm the traditional stereotype of the 'helpless epileptic'.

The extent to which social pressures affect the personality depends not only on the given temperament of the individual, but also on the environment in which he lives. Education, occupation, income, and class all play a part in determining how well or badly people with epilepsy survive the pressures they face. There are many studies of the personality of epileptics which show that it is their social background not their tendency to seizures that causes problems. According to one such study, epileptic children with personality disorders had, almost without exception, a poor home environment. Another study that compared the family situation of epileptic children with conduct disorders with epileptic children without conduct disorders and non-epileptic children with conduct disorders revealed that similar adverse factors (disturbed parental attitudes, marital disharmony, breaks and changes in the environment) were present in both conduct disorder groups, but not in the group of adjusted epileptic children.

Fits are responsible for personality changes in some people for several reasons. Many patients experience bouts of irritability and depression proceeding a fit; in other cases, a fit may evolve into a twilight state, during which the patient is confused and occasionally aggressive. But these mood-changes disappear once the fit has taken place and are rarely a permanent feature of the individual's personality.

Fits can also have a more indirect effect on the personality. There is probably a large number of epileptics who live in constant fear of having a seizure. It is not physical injury they are usually afraid of, but loss of self-esteem. They find it hard to accept that they could, at any time, lose control of themselves and, perhaps, act out of character. What they dread above all is the possibility of humiliation and of disapproval. The effect on the personality of such anxieties is hard to calculate, but is, no doubt, often damaging.

Personality problems are especially associated with temporal lobe epilepsy. A seizure discharge passing through one of the temporal lobes produces symptoms that often resemble those found in the mentally ill. Normally, these symptoms are confined to the fit, but sometimes they influence other aspects of a patient's life. During their seizures, people with temporal lobe epilepsy retain some degree of consciousness and are vaguely aware of the changes in their behaviour that are taking place. They see that it is *they* who are acting in an unusual manner, but, because their actions have not been willed, they also have the impression that they are no longer *themselves*. Patients sometimes speak of themselves as feeling disconnected, fragmented, malformed or incomplete during a temporal lobe seizure. In extreme cases, they may try to protect themselves from any further loss of self-identity by avoiding those situations in life that contain an element of emotional risk and by relying on habits and obsessions familiar enough to seem unthreatening. Such patients, in fact, adopt the rigid and inflexible characteristics that were once thought typical of the 'epileptic personality'.

Some anticonvulsants, notably phenobarbitone, phenytoin and primidone can produce personality changes ranging from mild confusion and irritability at one end of the spectrum to hallucinations and feelings of persecution at the other. Patients with temporal lobe epilepsy are particularly vulnerable in this respect. Aniticonvulsants have also been reported as causing behavioural problems in children with normal personalities, though these problems have cleared up as soon as the drugs have been withdrawn. Patients who take too many anti-epileptic drugs become drowsy. Sluggishness of thought and speech was often regarded as a typical epileptic trait in the days when bromides were administered in large quantities to patients to control their seizures.

One last point: mental illness is extremely common. In Britain each year an estimated 600,000 people seek psychiatric help. It would be amazing if a proportion of these did not also have epilepsy. But because some epileptics are mentally ill, is does not follow that their mental illness had been brought on by their having seizures.

Is There Any Connection Between Epilepsy and Crime?

A disproportionally large number of prisoners have epilepsy. Many of these people would be classed as socially inadequate. They have poor seizure control; possibly they suffer from some other neurological disorder in addition to epilepsy. For many of them, prison is the last refuge society has to offer. As usual, it would be illegitimate to generalize about all epileptics on the evidence of the most disabled, and there is no reason to think that most people with epilepsy are not as law-abiding as any other group of citizens.

A popular belief, one that seems to have originated in Victorian times, is that patients sometimes commit murder or rape during an epileptic seizure and are afterwards unaware of what they have done. There is little hard evidence to support this view. Some patients, especially men, act aggressively while in a state of automatism, but in a clumsy fashion, and without the concentration required to carry out an act of sustained violence. Crimes committed during automatisms tend to be minor — shoplifting, for example. Most epileptics in prison are there for theft and do not have any record of violence.

Patients who commit a serious crime during a fit can only use their epilepsy as a defence if they are prepared to plead not guilty by reason of insanity. If this plea is accepted, the judge has no option but to send the defendent to a secure hospital, where he will remain until such time as it is decided he is no longer a threat to the community. This is clearly unsatisfactory. Epileptic automatisms are not a form of insanity, but neither is a person fully in control of his actions during them. Either the courts should be given more discretion in these matters, or — better still — a plea of not guilty because of automatism (excluding alcoholic automatism) should be introduced.

Are there any Long-term Dangers in taking Anticonvulsant drugs?

Phenobarbitone has been used for the treatment of epilepsy since 1912, phenytoin since 1938 and primidone since 1952. The most recent anticonvulsant to be introduced, sodium valproate, has now been regularly prescribed in many different countries for over ten years. People with epilepsy probably take more drugs over a long period of time than any other kind of patient and anticonvulsants must, therefore, rank among the most thoroughly tested drugs in existence. Their side-effects are well-recognized. As such, it is possible to say, with some degree of certainty, that taking anticonvulsants over a period of time should not endanger a patient's health *providing he has his blood serum checked regularly and his drug levels adjusted in line with any changes in liver metabolism.*

Is It Safe for People with Epilepsy to Swim?

Keeping healthy is an important part of seizure-control, and everybody with epilepsy should make an effort to take regular exercise. Patients who have frequent seizures would be unwise to cycle on public roads and many would prefer to avoid contact sports, but providing they are well-supervised there is no reason why even those with poor seizure-control should not take exercise of some form or another. Swimming is an especially healthy activity; it strengthens the muscles and the cardio-vascular system and it improves co-ordination. There are probably few ways of keeping fit which are as enjoyable, as satisfactory or as useful as swimming. Its dangers to people with epilepsy have been exaggerated. Studies in Australia and Hawaii have shown that the risk of drowning as a result of an epileptic seizure is low. More people with epilepsy drown in their baths than they do at sea or in swimming pools, which is hardly surprising since most baths are taken in private.

People with epilepsy who wish to learn to swim should always practise under the supervision of a strong and capable swimmer, preferably someone who is a qualified life saver. Teachers should appoint a fellow pupil to companion an epileptic child when a class visits the local swimming pool. In this way, there is no chance of a fit passing unnoticed. Even experienced swimmers should never swim by themselves if there is a possiblity of them having a seizure.

When a person has an epileptic seizure in water, his swimming movements may briefly continue at first, then become unco-ordinated. He will start to splash and to lose direction and his head may begin to nod and roll. Life saving measures consist of keeping the head above water, and allowing the patient to breathe freely. He will do himself less harm if he has his fit in the water than if he is pulled ashore. After the fit is over, he should be helped onto dry land and left to recover in his own time in the usual way. Providing the patient has not injured himself, there is no need to call for medical assistance.

Does Having Epilepsy Shorten your Life?

Statistics collected by life insurance companies show that the mortality rate among people with epilepsy is two to three times greater than normal. Such overall figures, though, are misleading in so far as they do not distinguish between different types of epilepsy. Clearly, someone who suffers from a severe neurological disorder and who, in addition to having seizures, is mentally retarded and spastic will not have the same life expectancy as someone who, apart from having the occasional fit, is in good health.

Information about the mortality rate of people with epilepsy is derived mainly from death certificates. The way these are filled in varies from country to country and, to some extent, varies also between doctors in the same country, so that the difference between 'death due to epilepsy' and 'death of a person with epilepsy' is often blurred. Except for severe cases of status epilepticus, seizures are not, in themselves, life-threatening, although they can be a cause of death if the patient is driving a car or taking a bath when they happen.

The life expectancy of epileptics is related to the age of the individual. Children under the age of five have the highest mortality rate, followed in turn by people over the age of sixty-five and people aged between twenty-five and forty-five. Those who acquire the disease after the age of thirty have, statistically-speaking, a normal life expectancy. A person whose seizures are well-controlled and who otherwise is in good health stands much the same chance as any other healthy person of enjoying a normal lifespan. Progressive life insurance companies recognize this fact by charging many people with epilepsy normal, or only slightly-above normal, premiums.

9.

LIVING WITH EPILEPSY

Coming to Terms with Epilepsy

Patients respond in many different ways when they first learn they have epilepsy. Some become angry, blaming themselves or their parents or fate for what has happened. Some become depressed and see their future in the blackest of terms. Many are confused, uncertain, afraid. Few patients will have given the subject of epilepsy much thought until then and may be carrying all sorts of misconceptions round with them.

A patient's initial attitude will to a large extent be influenced by that of the doctor. If he is brusque, they may be unsure as to how serious epilepsy is. If he seems reluctant to answer their questions, thinking they will not understand what he says, they may imagine things are worse than they are. The doctor should make an effort to explain the facts to his patients. He should deal fully with their enquiries and encourage them to express their fears. Patients, for their part, should never feel their anxieties are too ridiculous or trivial to be discussed. An experienced doctor will almost certainly have come across every possible kind of response from his patients and is unlikely to be surprised by anything he is asked. Admittedly, some patients will only hear what they want to; but this is no excuse for the doctor not treating his patients as partners, entitled to learn the facts of their case, especially since it is the patients not the doctor who will be responsible for taking anticonvulsant drugs every day.

Often, the doctor will be unable to say what has caused a person to have seizures. This may be hard on those patients who feel that a disease without a known cause is like a detective story without an ending, but they should not, out of a feeling of dissatisfaction, be tempted into supplying a cause for themselves. There is little point in blaming one's epilepsy on some long-dead uncle who occasionally had a nervous tic; there is even less point in blaming one's self. Epilepsy is not a punishment for bad behaviour or unclean thoughts, but an organic disease, and there is no one who cannot develop it given the right circumstances.

These are general considerations. But what if it is *you* who are the patient? It may be more difficult then to be objective. The plain fact is, though, that if you are to make full use of your life and *control your seizures,* you must come to terms with the fact that you have epilepsy. Denial is a common response to unpleasant news, but not a very helpful one in the end. A neurologist will have seen so many cases of epilepsy during his career that there is little chance of you having been misdiagnosed. Accept first that you are subject to fits; only then can you do something about it.

If you find it difficult coming to terms with your epilepsy, this is probably because you see it as imposing unwelcome restrictions on your life. Seizures, you may feel, make you less free. They introduce an element of uncertainty into your affairs. They have been thrust upon you, not chosen. All this is true up to a point. But seizures are hardly the only thing in life over which we are not consulted. Normally, we are prepared to accept restrictions we know we cannot change. We adapt ourselves within the limits imposed on us, and do not usually consider our lives any poorer for that. Some degree of adaptation is also necessary in order to live with epilepsy, but not as much as many people think. There are many illnesses more disabling than epilepsy, illnesses that destroy the mind and the body. Epilepsy rarely prevents a person from living a normal life. Having seizures is often much less inconvenient than having asthma, arthritis or diabetes.

One of the first things you should do in order to come to terms with epilepsy is to learn a little about the disorder. As I have tried to show in this book, the facts about epilepsy are usually less alarming than the misconceptions. If you find yourself resisting the idea that you are subject to seizures, it is probably because you imagine the effects of seizures are worse than they are. You should realize that epilepsy:

— is neither an uncommon nor a fatal illness;

— does not lead to madness or an early death;

— does not usually grow worse with age, but on the contrary, often improves over a period of time;

— can be satisfactorily controlled in about 80 per cent of cases with drugs which, if administered properly, do not affect the mind or damage the body;

— is not a bar to marriage and is rarely a sufficient reason for not having children;

Most people with epilepsy are of normal intelligence and are able to live full lives. You are not a helpless victim. Your seizures do not control you; with modern medication, it is much more accurate to say that you control your seizures. The fact that you are reading this book is a sign that you have already taken the first steps towards coming to terms with your epilepsy.

Anticonvulsant Treatment

Always take the tablets you have been prescribed. As we saw in Chapter 6 a drug, once swallowed, is slowly broken down, till eventually the amount remaining in the blood is too small to have any measurable effect. It is necessary to keep the brain 'topped up' with an anticonvulsant drug; it is no good just taking a tablet when you feel like it. If you suddenly stop taking your tablets, you could have a status epilepticus fit — and that could be serious. You may feel, if you have gone without a seizure for a year or two, that you could manage on a lower dosage, or you may be worried that the drug you are taking is producing unpleasant side-effects. *Always* go and see your doctor if you have any queries like this. *Never* prescribe for yourself and *never* be tempted to try someone else's anticonvulsant drugs in exchange for yours. The doctor knows how long a drug takes to break down and what quantities you are taking, and he has asked you to take your tablets at certain specified times in order to ensure that there will always be a suffcent amount of the drug circulating in your bloodstream.*Always* keep to these times. Taking drugs too close together may overload the liver and cause poisioning; taking them too far apart puts you at risk of having a seizure.

If you have any problems remembering to take your tablets, try:

— making a note in a diary every time you take them. The effort of keeping a record will help reinforce your memory;

— linking tablet-taking with some well-established routine. Tablets which have to be taken three times a day can be swallowed after meals. If you have to take your tablets twice a day, then take one dose in the morning, on first rising or after breakfast, and the other dose with the evening meal, leaving about twelve hours in between;

— buying a small pillbox, which you should fill each evening with a day's supply of tablets. Take only the tablets in the pillbox, so that, by counting the number left you can tell how many you have already taken and whether you are due to take any more that day. Carry the pillbox with you if you expect to be out when you next need to take your tablets. So many people use drugs nowadays, for relieving headaches, mild depression and umpteen other minor complaints, that you shouldn't feel self-conscious about swallowing your tablets in public. If you cannot obtain a pillbox, a small medicine bottle will do almost as well, but make sure it is thoroughly cleaned out first.

Once tablet-taking has become a habit, you should have no problem remembering when to take them, nor will the taking of them seem quite the event it did when you first began your treatment.

Always make a point of learning the names of the tablets you have been prescribed and their strength (in milligrams). Apart from its practical value, such knowledge will help you overcome any sense you may have of being a passive victim blindly obeying incomprehensible orders dictated by fate and the doctor.

A Sensible Lifestyle

Apart from taking your anticonvulsants as prescribed, the best way to prevent seizures is to avoid any excess in your life. This doesn't mean being inflexible, a slave to routine. There is no reason why people with epilepsy should live a life devoid of adventure and challenge. But it is as well to observe a few sensible pre-cautions. Try not to overtax yourself, but take regular exercise and regular sleep, eat a balanced diet, keep your mind occupied. Don't mope or fret about the fact that you have epilepsy, or expect pity from others, and don't go around constantly worrying about having a seizure. Anxiety sometimes causes fits; there's no evidence that it ever prevents them.

Occasionally drinking a pint or two of beer, or one or two glasses of spirits or wine will probably do you no harm, but remember that, as someone with epilepsy and as a user of anticonvulsant drugs, you are doubly sensitive to the effects of alcohol; so don't overdo it. Carbamazepine slows down the rate at which water is excreted from the body. If you're taking this drug, you should avoid drinking large quantities of beer, or of any other liquid for that matter. Avoid alcohol altogether if you're on phenobarbitone: the two don't mix. Anatabuse, a drug which is given to alcoholics to wean them off drink, slows down the metabolic rate of the liver. Anyone who has epilepsy and is taking Anatabuse, will require smaller quantities of anticonvulsant drugs than before to achieve the same results.

If you have *frequent* seizures, you should;

— take showers, not baths. If you must have a bath, do not use more than about six inches of water, and leave the bathroom door unlocked in case you need help;

— leave the door unlocked when using the toilet. If you have a small WC, have a door fitted that opens outwards;

— cover open fires with guards, use safety racks on cookers etc.;

— avoid climbing on stepladders and chairs, or do so only if there is someone with you;

— carry an identity card with you when you go out. The card should contain your name and address and the name and address of your doctor, instructions to passers-by about what to do (and not do) during a fit and a note as to how long it normally takes you to recover consciousness. The British Epilepsy Association issue free identity cards to all their members. Stainless steel bracelets and necklaces can be purchased from the Medic-Alert Foundation. When you become a member of the Foundation, your name and medical details are entered on a central file in London and the Foundation's telephone number and the word Epilepsy are engraved on the bracelet. Information about you is only given out in an emergency and then only to doctors and to other authorized persons;

— if you are sometimes incontinent during a seizure, avoid drinking large quantities of liquid, go to the toilet regularly and put a waterproof sheet on top of your mattress.

— if you have reflex epilepsy, try and stay clear of any stimulus that might provoke a seizure. On sunny days, people with photosensitive epilepsy should wear polaroid sunglasses. Ordinary tinted spectacles will not give protection from the effects of flicker.

— if you have nocturnal epilepsy, use a non-suffocating pillow on your bed.

Mothers with epilepsy should observe a few simple rules to avoid the danger of dropping their child, or letting it put itself at risk, during a fit. So:

— don't wash the baby in a bath. Instead place the baby on a mat in its cot and wash it with water from a bowl placed on the outside of the bars;

— breast-feed the baby while lying on the bed, or — to be safer still — sit on the floor with your back to the wall. Then, if you have a seizure, you will most likely slide sidewards;

— when bottle feeding, strap the baby into its chair; it is also safer to strap the baby to the chair when moving it around the house, rather than to hold it in your arms;

— put gates on the kitchen door and on the stairs; fix a guard to the cooker to prevent pans being pulled off the hob; see the garden is well-fenced; keep doors shut and store your tablets out of reach of children.

Parents of Children with Epilepsy

Much of what has been said about the patient also applies to parents of children with epilepsy. Their reaction, on first learning that their child has epilepsy, like that of the patient, will probably consist of a mixture of uncertainty, surprise, distress, anger, guilt and depression. As with the patient it is essential, if they are to come to terms with their child's condition, to pass through this initial stage and to achieve a more realistic understanding of what it means to have seizures. There is a tendency for some parents to think that special skills are required to bring up a child with epilepsy. Certainly, they must ensure that their child never fails to receive his anticonvulsant drugs, that he is protected from any situations that might cause him to have a seizure, and that he doesn't take any unnecessary risks with his health. But unless their child has exceptionally poor seizure control this is likely to be the full extent of their nursing duties.

If you are a parent in this situation you should:

— try and overcome any sense of disgust or pity you may feel when you see your child having a fit. Don't be ashamed if these are your reactions — they are common enough — but realize that they don't serve any purpose and are almost certainly rooted in a false view of the nature of epilepsy;

— don't regard your child as a burden on your life or as a potential source of social embarrassment because he has fits. Never try to hide him away for fear of what relatives or neighbours might say if they see him having a seizure. Treating epilepsy as something shameful will only make your child feel inadequate;

— don't overprotect your child. Difficult as it may be to accept, it is far better for him to have an occasional seizure than to be prevented from taking part in normal activities. Unless there are sound medical reasons to the contrary, he should be allowed to take part in sports, play with his friends, visit their homes and do everything that a healthy non-epileptic child would do.

Cocooning him from the bruising effects of life will not only make him feel freakish, but will ill-prepare him for the future. Sooner or later, the time will come when he will leave home and mix with people who are not prepared to make the same allowances for him as you have done. The realization that having epilepsy does not entitle a person to special privileges can come as a terrible shock to anyone who has been brought up to think otherwise. Don't spoil your child from a misplaced sense of his own fragility. Spoilt children can manipulate their parents mercilessly, throwing temper tantrums and threatening to have a fit whenever they are crossed. Other children in a family naturally resent it if a brother or sister is always being favoured above them;

— never allow your child's epilepsy to so dominate your life that you have no time left for your partner;

— never use your child's epilepsy as an excuse to explain away his rudeness, deceitfulness, selfishness or any other kind of behaviour you disapprove of. Doing so not only creates the false impression that there is something 'bad' about epilepsy, but will also be resented by your child who will feel — rightly — that he is being judged by a different set of standards from everyone else. Certainly, you need to be aware that your child's behaviour could be affected by poor seizure-control or excessive medication, but where there is no evidence that either of these are involved, then telling him that it is not he but his epilepsy that is responsible for his actions is simply insulting;

— keep fits in their proper perspective. Don't treat them as if they were a tragedy, for they aren't. Don't panic when they happen. Don't keep reminding your child that he has epilepsy. Don't use the threat of a seizure as a means of restraining him whenever you want his compliance. Do nothing, in fact, to make the child resent having epilepsy;

— make an effort to learn something about the nature of epilepsy;

— offer your child regular and generous doses of praise and encouragement — as any good parent would.

Some young children have difficulty in swallowing their anticonvulsant tablets. Often it helps to crush the tablet first and then to mix it with the child's food, or to give it to him in a spoonful of honey or jam. If these tactics fail, you should consult your doctor who may be able to prescribe the same drug in a syrup or liquid (suspension) form, or as a chewable tablet. Drugs which are served in a suspension tend to separate out from the filler and sink to the bottom of the bottle when left to stand. It is important always to shake the bottle before use, otherwise each spoonful of the liquid may not contain the same amount of the drug.

Children with television epilepsy need not be prevented from watching television providing a few simple precautions are taken. There should always be a small illuminated table lamp on top of the set, which should be viewed in a well-lit room from a distance of at least eight feet. The child should never be allowed to flick rapidly from station to station and should only approach the set after first placing a hand over one eye as this cuts down the number of retinal cells stimulated by the flickering picture. Defective sets should be turned off (if necessary with the plug removed) until they are repaired.

Young children generally find it easier to accept their epilepsy than do older children and adults, perhaps because they have fewer expectations of what life should be like. Some interest in their own fits may be detectable in children round about the age of four, although at this stage it will probably be enough for them to know that their occasional lapses of consciousness have a name. Introducing them to the words 'fits' or 'black-outs' may be all that is needed in the way of education. As the child grows older, he will want to know more about what happens when he has a seizure, and why he has them, and whether he will stop having them in the future. Parents, having first acquainted themselves with the facts, should make every effort to answer their child's questions. Should they refuse to, the child is likely to think that things are worse than they are. Withholding the truth from him will not dampen his curiosity, but will simply make him more prepared to accept some of the misconceptions about epilepsy freely available in every school playground. Parents who wish to tell their child about his epilepsy, but who doubt their ability to explain a difficult subject in simple words, should at least offer him some suitable literature to read. There are a number of good books on the market, covering all age ranges, that deal with the subject in the form of an entertaining story, and if your local library has none of these, you should write to the British Epilepsy Association, who will supply you with a list of titles.

The British Epilepsy Association
This is an organization that everyone who has epilepsy, or who

has a child with epilepsy, should join. Founded in 1950, the BEA:

— provides professional advice and counselling for patients and their families and for employers, and offers back-up support through a network of self-help groups;

— publishes a comprehensive range of literature, much of it free;

— helps, through its Epilepsy Research fund, to promote research into the medical and social aspects of epilepsy;

— stages conferences, seminars and lectures for both professional and lay audiences and generally works to improve the general public's understanding of epilepsy; and

— represents people with epilepsy at appeal and industrial tribunals and acts as an intermediary between employers and their workers in disputes connected with epilepsy.

In return for a small membership fee (£5 a year at the time of writing), members receive free accident insurance, a quarterly newsletter, *Epilepsy Now!* and free literature about different aspects of epilepsy, as well as the other benefits offered by the Association. An important part of the £400,000 needed every year to maintain the BEA's facilities is raised by members through the Action for Epilepsy campaign. The local self-help groups provide people with epilepsy with the opportunity to discuss their problems with others in a similar position to themselves.

Conclusion
Much still remains to be learnt about epilepsy and, no doubt, in the future new and better forms of treatment will be discovered. But, already enough is known for us to say with certainty that epilepsy is not the horrific disease popular superstition pictures it as being, and that most patients can — and do —live full and active lives in spite of their fits. Over the last century the study of epilepsy has become a sophisticated enterprise. By comparison, social attitudes towards epilepsy are, in many instances, only just emerging from the Dark Ages. The urgent need now is not for some scientific breakthrough but for a better understanding by the public that people with epilepsy are people first and epileptics second. Only when the facts about epilepsy become more widely-known will this understanding be achieved.

GLOSSARY

Absence seizure: A *generalized* fit characterized by a momentary loss of consciousness; a petit mal.

Alpha rhythm: The normal EEG rhythm of the conscious adult brain during moments of inattention.

Amnesia: Loss of memory. A common side-effect of head injury. The inability to remember events immediately preceeding loss of consciousness is known as retrograde amnesia.

Anoxia: Deficiency of oxygen in the blood.

Artery: A type of blood vessel. Arteries carry oxygen-rich blood away from the heart. Blood is transported back to the heart through the veins.

Ataxia: Lack of muscular co-ordination such as is found in many kinds of drug intoxication.

Audiogenic seizure: Seizures provoked by sound; a type of *reflex epilepsy.*

Aura: A *motor* or *sensory seizure* of focal origin that preceeds a generalized seizure.

Attention: The process of being aware of, and of concentrating on, ideas, objects, people or events.

Axon: A part of the *neuron;* a fibre that carries the nerve impulse away from the neuron.

Beta rhythm: The normal EEG rhythm of the conscious adult brain during moments of *attention* (cf. *alpha rhythm*).

Carotid artery: An *artery,* situated either side of the neck, that carries most of the blood to the brain.

Central nervous system: The brain and spinal cord; the part of the nervous system responsible for co-ordinating the activities of the body.

Clonic seizure: A seizure in which the muscles alternately relax and contract.

Complex seizure: A type of *focal* fit characterized by distortions of memory, thought or emotion and often accompanied by motor or sensory symptoms.

Dendrite: A part of the *neuron;* dendrites carry the nerve impulse to the neuron (cf. *axon*).

Electroencephalogram: A recording of the changes in electrical activity of the neurons near the surface of the brain; a brain wave tracing.

Encephalitis: Inflammation of the brain resulting from an infection.

Epileptic focus: The area in the brain from which a *seizure discharge* originates.

Excitation: The process whereby a cell or a group of cells is stimulated into activity; the opposite of *inhibition.*

Febrile convulsion; A form of seizure, brought on by a fever, that affects young children.

Focal epilepsy: A type of epilepsy caused by a *lesion* in one cerebral hemisphere; partial epilepsy.

Foetus: The offspring in the mother's womb from about the third month until birth. Before this age it is known as an embryo.

Gene: The part of the chromosome that tranmits data from one generation to the next; the basic unit of heredity. A dominant gene is one whose effects appear in the offspring irrespective of whether or not it is matched with a like gene from the chromosome of the other mate. The effects of a recessive gene only appear when matched by a like gene.

Generalized epilepsy: A form of epilepsy in which both cerebral hemispheres are simultaneously affected by the seizure discharge. Generalized seizures can either be *primary* or *secondary.*

Glia cell; A type of nerve cell. Its function is to protect and nourish the *neuron..*

Hormone: A chemical substance released into the bloodstream by a gland in order to influence the action of other organs.

Idiopathic epilepsy: Any form of epilepsy whose cause is unknown.

Inhibition; The opposite of *excitation.*

Jacksonian seizure: A form of focal motor seizure which begins in one muscle, or set of muscles, and gradually extends over larger areas in a march-like fashion.

Lesion: Any localized injury.

Meninges: Three layers of tissue that cover the brain and spinal cord. Between two of the layers are spaces filled with cerebro-spinal fluid.

Meningitis: Inflammation of the meninges resulting from infection.

Metabolism; The process, or processes, by which substances are converted in the body from one form to another.

Motor seizure; A seizure originating in the motor cortex; any fit involving the muscles.

Myoclonic seizure: A form of *motor seizure* consisting of brief, shock-like jerks of the limbs and/or the trunk.

Neurology: The scientific study of the nervous system.

Neuron: The nerve cell; the part of the nervous system that generates the nerve impulse. Sometimes spelt neurone.

Partial epilepsy: Focal epilepsy.

Photogenic seizure: A form of reflex seizure provoked by flashing light; a photosensitive fit.

Primary generalized epilepsy: A type of *generalized epilepsy* that originates simultaneously in both cerebral hemispheres. Usually regarded as being genetically-acquired.

Secondary generalized epilepsy: A type of *generalized epilepsy* that begins in one cerebral hemisphere as a focal seizure before crossing over into the other hemisphere.

Seizure discharge: A nerve discharge, arising from an *epileptic focus,* that disrupts brain activity and manifests itself in the form of an epileptic fit.

Sensory seizure: A seizure originating in one of the sensory areas in the brain and characterized by alterations in vision, taste, feeling etc., according to the area involved.

Status epilepticus: A condition in which one fit follows another with little or no recovery in between.

Symptomatic epilepsy: Any form of epilepsy whose cause is known.

*Term assurance:*A form of Life Assurance. The policy holder is paid an agreed sum on the death of the person insured.

Tonic seizure: A fit in which the muscles tighten and become rigid.

Trauma: Any severe injury, particularly one involving the skull.

Twilight state: A confused state following on a seizure.

Whole assurance: A form of Life Assurance. As with *term assurance,* the policy holder receives a sum of money on the death of the insured person, but, in addition, also receives a proportion of the premiums paid towards the policy. Because of the investment content, premiums are charged at a higher rate for whole than for term assurance.

USEFUL ADDRESSES

The British Epilepsy Association

Head Office:

Crowthorne House,
Bigshotte,
New Wokingham Road,
WOKINGHAM,
Berkshire RG11 3AY
(0344 773122)

Regional Offices:

313 Chapeltown Road,
LEEDS LS7 3JT
(0532 621076)

1st Floor — Guildhall Bldgs.,
Navigation Street,
BIRMINGHAM B2 4BT
(021-643 7740)

178 Whitchurch Road,
CARDIFF CF4 3NB
(0222 628744)

The Old Postgraduate Medical,
Belfast City Hospital,
BELFAST BT9 7AB
(0232 248414)

The Mersey Region Epilepsy Association

138 The Albany,
Old Hall Street,
LIVERPOOL L3 9EY
(051-236 0990)

The Epilepsy Association of Scotland

Head Office:

48 Govan Road,
GLASGOW G51 1JL.
(041-427 4911)

Regional Offices:

13 Guthrie Street,
EDINBURGH EH1 1JG.
(031-226 5458)

35 Woodmuir Terrace,
NEWPORT ON TAY.
(0382 21545)

The National Society for Epilepsy

Chalfont Centre for Epilepsy
Chalfont St. Peter,
GERRARDS CROSS,
Buckinghamshire SL9 0RJ.
(02407 3991)
Provides a valuable information service.

The International Bureau for Epilepsy

PO Box 21,
2100 AA Heemstede,
THE NETHERLANDS
(010-31-23-339060)

For details about foreign epilepsy associations.

Schools and Centres for Epilepsy

Chalfont Centre for Epilepsy
(see previous page)

David Lewis Centre & School
Warford,
Near ALDERLEY EDGE,
Cheshire
(056-587 2153)

Cookridge Hall,
Ridgeside,
Cookridge,
LEEDS LS16 7NL.
(0532 673448)

St. Elizabeth's School & Home,
South End,
MUCH HADHAM,
Hertfordshire.
(027-984 2233)

Lingfield Hospital School,
LINGFIELD,
Surrey,
(0342 832243)

The Maghull Homes,
MAGHULL,
Near Liverpool L31 8BR.
(051-526 4133)

The Meath Home for Epileptic
Women & Girls,
GODALMING,
Surrey.
(04868 5095)

Quarrier's Homes,
BRIDGE OF WEIR,
Renfrewshire.
(0505-61 2224)

Insurance

Tyser & Co. Ltd.,
Ellerman House,
12-20 Camomile Street,
LONDON EC3A 7PJ.
(01-623 6262)

Driving Licence Applications

DVLC,
SWANSEA SA99 1AB.
(0792 72151)

The Medic-Alert Foundation

11-13 Clifton Terrace,
LONDON N4 3JP.
(01-263 8597)

FURTHER READING

There are a number of books on epilepsy written for lay readers. Two of the best are *Epilepsy: The Facts* by Anthony Hopkins (Oxford University Press, 1984) and *About Epilepsy* by Donald Scott (Duckworth, 1981). *The Epilepsy Reference Book* by Peter M. Jeavons and Alec Aspinal (Harper and Row, 1985) is also recommended. The practical aspects of epilepsy are dealt with in *The Epilepsy Handbook* by Shelagh McGovern (Sheldon Press, 1982) and *People with Epilepsy* by Mary B. Laidlaw and John Laidlaw (Churchill Livingstone, 1984).

Two good introductions to neurology, both published by Penguin Books, are *The Nervous System* by Peter Nathan (1969) and *The Conscious Brain* by Steven Rose (1976). *Understanding EEG* by Donald Scott (Duckworth, 1976) is very accessible. Short essays on different aspects of epilepsy are featured in *Epilepsy '78, Epilepsy '79* and *Perspectives on Epilepsy 80/1* published by the British Epilepsy Association.

Oswei Temkin has written a fascinating history of epilepsy entitled *The Falling Sickness* (John Hopkins University Press, 1971). *A Ray of Darkness* by Margiad Evans (John Calder, 1978) is the autobiography of a woman with epilepsy. Younger readers may be interested in *What Difference Does It Make, Danny?*, a story about a child who has fits, written by Helen Young and illustrated by Quentin Blake. Copies are available from the British Epilepsy Association.

Probably the most comprehensive work on epilepsy is W. G. Lennox's two volume *Epilepsy and Related Disorders* (Little, Brown and Co., 1960). Although written primarily for specialists, Lennox's book is often very readable. A more up-to-date, but drier, account of the subject is contained in *A Textbook of Epilepsy* edited by John Laidlaw and Alan Richens (Churchill Livingstone,

1980). *The Epilepsies* by John M. Sutherland and Mervyn J. Eadie (Churchill Livingstone, 1980) is short and succinct. *Anticonvulsant Therapy* by Mervyn J. Eadie and John H. Tyrer (Churchill Livingstone, 1980) and *Comprehensive Management of Epilepsy in Infancy, Childhood and Adolescence* by Samuel Livingston (Charles C. Thomas, 1972) are both standard works. Extensive details about the relationship between the brain and seizures will be found in *Epilepsy and the Functional Anatomy of the Human Brain* by Wilder Penfield and Herbert Jasper (Little, Brown and Co., 1954).

INDEX